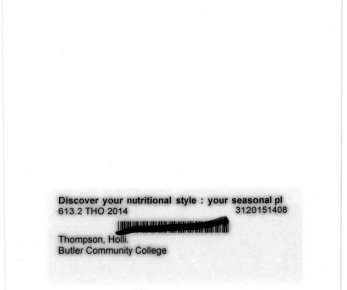

Discover your nutritional style : your seasonal pl
613.2 THO 2014   3120151408

Thompson, Holli.
Butler Community College

Additional Praise

■ Holli Thompson presents the cornerstone of modern nutrition, flexibility, in a very easy to read and visually appealing book. Although there are many dietary philosophies, the end goal for all of them remains the same: a better and longer life. This book is a good start on that lifelong journey.
— **BARRY SEARS, PhD**, Author of *The Zone*, President of the Inflammation Research Foundation

■ Holli Thompson's book, *Discover Your Nutritional Style*, is an outstanding example of what a Certified Holistic Health Coach trained by INN does for her clients and readers. Holli provides the information and support you need to discover your personal Nutritional Style. You'll learn to eat in a flexible, holistic way that's right for you all year-round.
— **JOSHUA ROSENTHAL**, Founder and Director of the Institute for Integrative Nutrition

■ *Discover Your Nutritional Style* is the perfect guide to a holistic eating approach. It helps you to create the perfect connection between the foods you eat and how you feel, season by season. Holli's passion comes from her own health struggles and her willingness to support everyone along the way. This book is a must read! It's the LBD (Little Black Dress) for your Nutritional Style. I'm all about fitting into my Little Black Dress, no matter what season.
— **MICHELLE KING ROBSON**, Founder of EmpowHER.com

■ With *Discover Your Nutritional Style*, Holli Thompson has created an extraordinary tool. She's distilled her unique coaching experience and tons of great information into a book that encourages a collaborative process with the reader. Her emphasis on helping you find your own style (rather than offering a cookie-cutter solution that simply doesn't fit you) means that you will wind up with a plan that reflects your own needs, behaviors, and desires, and makes it easy for you to change your life.
— **JOE CROSS**, Author of *Reboot with Joe*, Founder of rebootwithjoe.com

■ Holli Thompson's *Discover Your Nutritional Style* is a beautifully crafted book that deserves to be on the shelf of anyone interested in food and health. Get ready for a feast of great information, practical tips, and surprising insights. Whereas so many nutrition books seem to hit us over the head with hard-to-follow do's and don'ts, Holli has a warm and inviting approach that'll leave you inspired to make changes in your kitchen, your body, and your life. Highly recommended.
— **MARC DAVID**, Founder of the Institute for the Psychology of Eating

■ In *Discover Your Nutritional Style*, Holli Thompson dishes up a nourishing dose of nutritional guidance with style, grace, and humor. More than just a book on healthy eating, Holli will feel like your best girlfriend and coach rolled into one as she teaches you how to choose your personal path to a happier, healthier you. Highly recommended!
— **JAN NEUHARTH**, Author of the *Hunt Country Suspense* novels

■ Holli knows that diet is a lot like religion; it's not one-size-fits-all. Her brilliant insight helps the reader navigate the changing landscape of food and health that we find ourselves on today. This book is such a valuable tool for 21st-century eaters.

— **ROBYN O'BRIEN,** Founder of AllergyKids Foundation, Author of *The Unhealthy Truth*

■ *Discover Your Nutritional Style* is a fantastic book for anyone interested in health. It is approachable, full of excellent information, and most important, encourages you to pursue the diet that is best for your body.

— **MAX GOLDBERG,** Founder of maxgoldberg.com, Creator of pressedjuicedirectory.com

■ Holli's book wisely and *beautifully* inspires us to transform our diets based on the season and style of Mother Nature herself. Wherever you live on this lovely planet of ours, Holli's recommendations and recipes are a simple, yet profound guide to using the power of seasonal foods.

— **ALEX JAMIESON,** Author of *The Great American Detox Diet*

■ If readers have struggled with healthy intentions—unsuccessfully—Holli's book provides new hope, opening the door for a journey of inspiring, creative, healthful strategies.

— **BILL COUZENS**, Founder of Less Cancer, lesscancer.org

■ Holli meets people where they are, in their diet and nutrition, and inspires them to be better, happier, and healthier. *Discover Your Nutritional Style* does all that and more, with real-life ways on how to achieve your ideal health, beginning with helping you discover your Nutritional Style. Plus a smart way to detox, the bad-boys of nutrition, and a seasonal approach to food and eating that I love, especially the raw foods!

— **SARMA MELNGAILIS**, Author of *Living Raw Food*, Owner of Pure Food and Wine restaurant, NYC

■ *Discover Your Nutritional Style* is a winner! Holli sets us free from strict rules and the angst many of us feel around eating. She delivers a simple and seasonal way to eat that's uniquely designed to unleash your highest levels of health, happiness, and vitality. Get this book now.

— **MARIE FORLEO,** Award Winning Host of MarieTV, MarieForleo.com.

■ I'm a big believer that the best foods to eat are different for everyone. Holli does a great job in *Discover Your Nutritional Style,* making it easy and fun to find the best foods for you and your body.

— **JARED KOCH**, Founder and Co-Author of *Clean Plates*

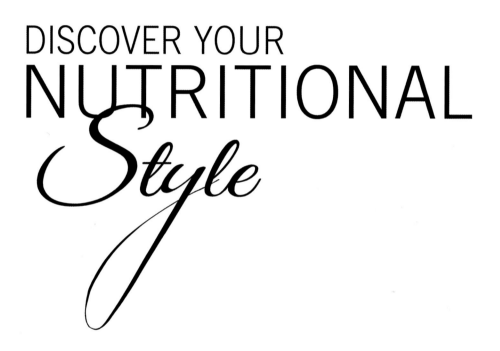

DISCOVER YOUR NUTRITIONAL *Style*

DISCOVER YOUR
NUTRITIONAL
Style

Your Seasonal Plan
to a Healthy, Happy
and Delicious Life

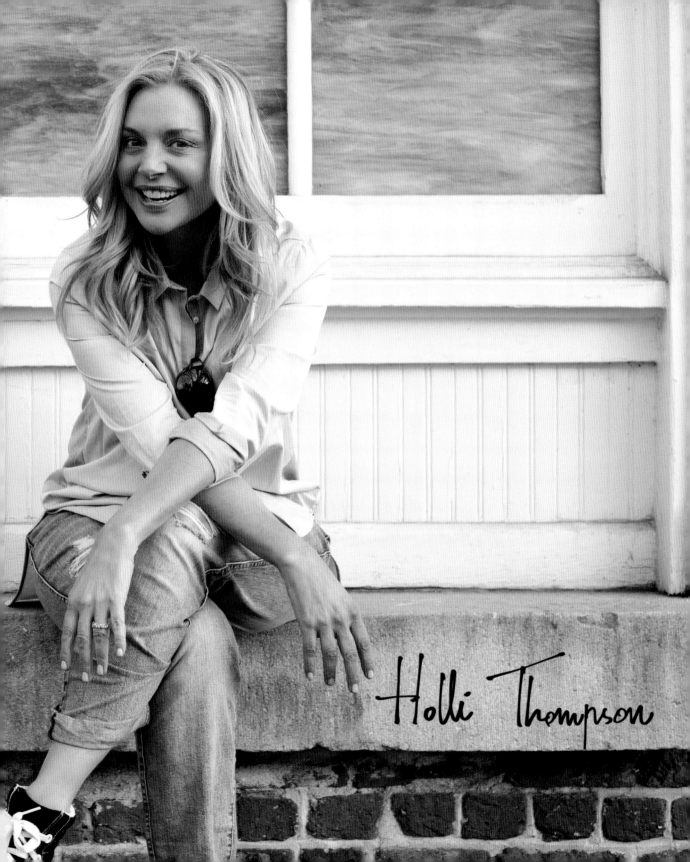

Holli Thompson

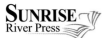

Sunrise River Press
39966 Grand Avenue
North Branch, MN 55056
Phone: 651-277-1400 or 800-895-4585
Fax: 651-277-1203
www.sunriseriverpress.com

Edit: Sheila Buff
Layout: Connie DeFlorin
Cover design: Connie DeFlorin
Cover photography: Chelsea Fullerton/Go Forth Creative
Food photography: Chelsea Fullerton/Go Forth Creative
Art direction: Jennifer Elsner/Viewers Like You
Photo styling: Jennifer Elsner/Viewers Like You
Illustrations: Marta Spendowska/verymarta.com

ISBN 978-1-934716-44-1
Item No. SRP644

Library of Congress Cataloging-in-Publication Data

Thompson, Holli.
  Discover your nutritional style / by Holli Thompson.
     pages cm
  ISBN 978-1-934716-44-1
  1. Nutrition--Popular works. 2. Food habits--Popular
works. 3. Detoxification (Health) 4. Health behavior--Pop-
ular works. 5. Self-care, Health--Popular works. I. Title.
  RA784.T529 2014
  613.2--dc23
                                    2014006250

Written, edited, and designed in the U.S.A.
Printed in China

10 9 8 7 6 5 4 3 2 1

Dedication

I dedicate this book to my parents, Margaret and Joseph Perone,
who taught me that good food is worth all the effort.

For Moses and Ormsby.

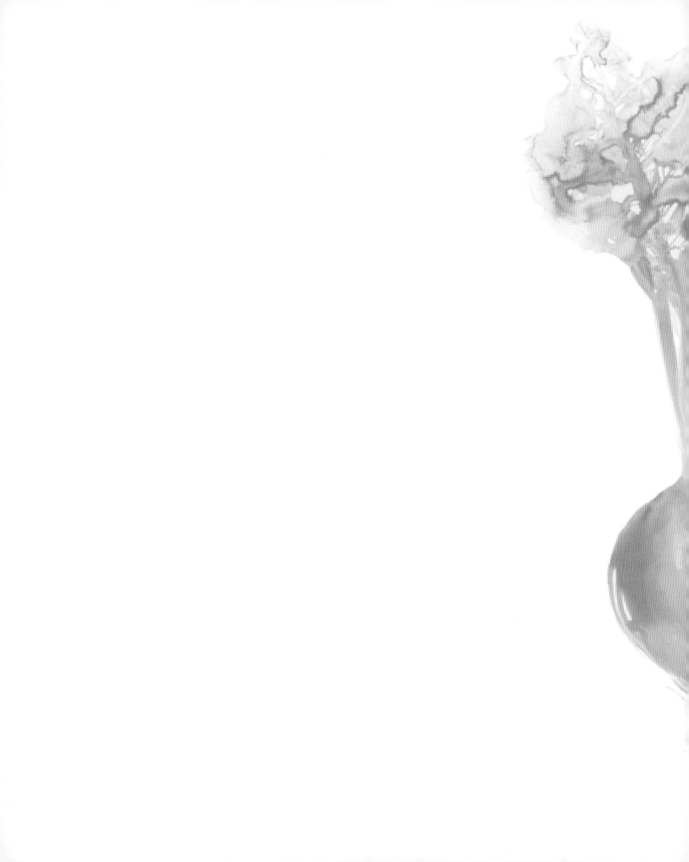

Contents

Foreword

by Frank Lipman, MD

I n my practice, I often treat people who aren't as healthy as they want to be. They feel tired, worn-out, not quite right. They get frequent infections, headaches, and digestive upsets. They have so little energy that they feel older than their chronological age.

They come to me because they want their health and energy back. Once I'm sure they don't have anything medically wrong with them, I work with my patients to renew their capacity for a vital, active life.

A crucial first step is to look at a patient's diet, because what we eat has a profound effect on how we feel. For many of my patients, years of unbalanced eating turns out to be a major part of their constant exhaustion and poor functioning.

When we start talking about diet, many patients insist that they eat well. When we talk more, however, it's clear that they don't eat well at all. In fact, between trendy diets and all the dietary misinformation that floats around in magazine articles and online, they've often ended up eating in ways that are often just wrong for them despite their best intentions.

Every person is different. A diet that works well for one person may be completely wrong for someone else. And even a diet that works well for you now may not work as well at a different time of year, or when your life circumstances change.

That's why I'm so glad to be writing this foreword to Holli Thompson's *Discover Your Nutritional Style.* Holli knows, from her own experience and from her training and experience as a health coach, how vital it is to craft a diet that is right for you. More important, she understands that things change. The style that keeps you feeling well-fed and healthy may change as you change.

Holli has often worked with me to coach participants through my cleansing process. I know from my own experience that she truly understands the value of doing a safe, gentle cleanse as a way to renew your body and shake off the effects of the toxins that surround us and the toxic effects of stress. Cleansing isn't always easy, and Holli is wonderful at helping people solve their issues with it. She's even better at encouraging them to make the long-term dietary changes that help them stick with a healthier lifestyle.

Holli is a creative problem-solver and an empathetic, well-trained health coach. I'm delighted that she's written a book that incorporates her ideas and her enthusiasm. Use this book to discover your own Nutritional Style and learn to lead a happier and healthier life.

Acknowledgments

Thank you from my heart to:

My clients and community. Thank you for believing that I had something to offer and for your trust, confidence, and support. I am grateful and blessed to have you.

Sunrise River Press, most especially to Molly Koecher for discovering me in *More* magazine and for overseeing this book with such care. I am grateful.

More magazine Editor-in-Chief Lesley Jane Seymour, for highlighting my work as a Reinvention Story in her magazine.

My guest contributors: Dr. Mark Hyman, Sarma Melngailis, Natalia Rose, Dr. Alejandro Junger, Jenny Nelson, Elizabeth Petty, and Amy Waldman. Most especially to Dr. Frank Lipman, for writing the foreword, and to Jennifer Mielke.

Joshua Rosenthal and the team at the Institute for Integrative Nutrition for leading the way and changing my life.

Sheila Buff, for your nutritional wisdom and incredible editing talent.

Jennifer Elsner, for your impeccable sense of design, beauty, and style for my overall brand; for creating my website; and for your influence, design direction, and styling. To Chelsea Fullerton, for your talented and inspiring photography. Your great eye, infectious laugh, and lovely persona made it all fun, casual, and easy.

To the photo shoot team: Thank you to the Ellwood Thompson stores for allowing us a beautiful and healthy location. More location thank-yous to Bill Sorrell and Rob Smith, Michelle Martello, and Jennifer Elsner and David Shields for allowing us access to your homes. To Lauren Thorsen for her production skills, and to Jennifer Saunders and Mary Dandridge, the two styling angels.

Robin Colucci, for coaxing this book out of me, with so much gratitude.

Pamela Henning, for being a wonderful, supportive friend from the very beginning.

Bill Couzens, for founding Less Cancer, being a great friend, and making me laugh.

Karin Witzig Rozell, Leni Onkka, Erika Lyremark, Nisha Moodley, Tara Sophia Mohr, Danielle LaPorte, and Marie Forleo, for your wisdom and inspirational coaching.

Janice Formicella, for your research, support, and everything else.

My girlfriends—you know who you are. Thank you for listening and cheering me on. I love you ladies and could not have written this book without your help; dragging me out of the house, encouraging me to keep going, and making me laugh.

My mastermind and entrepreneur colleagues, we're in this together, and I'm so happy to be in your circle.

Mom and Dad, I love you and I am grateful to be your daughter, and thank you to my sisters and your families for your support.

My son, Nathanael Ormsby Nikolai Anatoly Thompson. I'm sorry my head was buried in my Mac so much this past year(s). Thank you for being you.

Moses, I will always be yours. Thank you for listening and being there for me.

And to my adopted furry companions, who are by my side each day.

From Down and Out to Discovering My Nutritional Style

I'm a health and nutrition coach, a certified natural health practitioner, and to make it fun, a nutrition stylist. The stylist part is my nod to my "glamorous" past life as an executive in the fashion and fine jewelry industry. (Anyone who's ever worked in fashion knows the glamour part is way overrated, but that's another story.)

As a coach, I work mainly with women, many of them entrepreneurs, most of them in their thirties or older. It's a time fraught with hormonal changes, aging issues, energy issues. As I like to say, it's the time in life when you reap what you have sown. It's when you realize you can no longer get away with eating whatever is in front of you. The women I work with want to feel fabulous every day, they want to live life as beautifully as possible, and they want to take their family and partners along for the ride.

I work with these women to help them find their own Nutritional Style. Through food, we change their lives. We go back to the nutritional basics and take a holistic approach to eating and living, one that's connected to the seasons and all they have to offer.

The people I coach are often successful, hard-working, and overachievers. They're passionate about their lives, but sometimes they need help understanding their own needs. My clients are *so* competent they think they're infallible—until they start to look older, or every meal upsets their digestion, or until aches and pains or a lack of energy forces them to take a look at their lifestyle and their food.

Fashion Exec to Mom to Health Coach

I can help these women understand how and why they need to change their diets because I was one of them.

I was in my midthirties, single, and a vice president for Chanel, with an office overlooking Central Park and a clothing allowance that kept me in head-to-toe Chanel—including the handbags. I helped develop and then launched Chanel's fine jewelry and watch division; it was an amazing career. I traveled back and forth to Paris and worked with incredibly talented people. I absolutely loved my life and my job. I couldn't have designed anything more fun or more perfect for me at the time.

Then I met my husband. He lived in Virginia, and had his own company, a young daughter, and lots of responsibilities. It was love at first sight—well, maybe first lunch—and the dear friend who'd introduced us was shocked. She didn't intend for us to fall in love and get married within eight months.

Each weekend, I traveled back and forth from New York City to his idyllic home in the Virginia countryside surrounded by acres of fields, horses, cows, and more horses and cows. We started riding every weekend. My instant mom status was a lot of fun and very quickly became an important part of my life.

After about a year or so doing the weekend commute, our first fine jewelry collection for Chanel launched successfully. Needless to say, by then I was tired. The travel was getting to me, and switching between big city fashion executive during the week and country step-mom on the weekends made my life seem too disparate. I realized one day that in a year of marriage, my husband and I had never spent more than five days together at a time. A change was needed.

I sadly resigned from Chanel, leaving the best job in the world. I shipped my furniture and piled dozens of overstuffed garment bags into my new husband's SUV, along with two fancy city cats who could not imagine where their new life would lead. Get ready, city cats, this'll rock your world.

I loved living with my husband (I guess that's always a good thing!), but living in the country full-time was a challenge. I hadn't yet made friends, and I was lonely. As someone who'd been working since age 12, I decided I finally needed some time off. My husband suggested that maybe some self-exploration was in order.

Wow, time to think? That would be new.

I signed up for painting classes and bought a horse. I started running every day for miles on dirt roads, hung out at the barn where we boarded my mare, and spent most of my time alone. It was a big change, but I was happily in love and sure that my new passion and career were on their way.

That was true, but I had no idea how painful the process would be.

One day a few months later, we took my stepdaughter and her cousins to a horse show. It was early June in Virginia, and the heat was over 100, with high humidity. I was worried the kids would overheat, so I pushed them to drink more water. I forgot about myself.

Suddenly, while sitting in the sun with the children dancing around me, I got a searingly painful headache. I managed to stand and murmur to my husband, "Please get me out of here."

My head was splitting in two, I was dizzy and nauseous, and I needed my husband to hold me up as we staggered to our car. I tried to play it down so I wouldn't scare the children, but by the time we reached our house I was unable to walk.

A friend decided I must be dehydrated and went out to buy electrolyte drinks. I lay in bed thinking I was going to die. An hour later, the pain was so severe I could no longer speak or move. My husband called an ambulance.

I stayed in the hospital for days while the doctors ran every test possible. The pain was unbearable; I was on a morphine drip to keep it at bay.

The frustrating part was that no one could say what was wrong. There was no diagnosis, although one doctor, after hearing about my drastic switch from high-powered VP to country mom, did venture to say, "Some people aren't meant to retire." I remember wanting to slug him, but instead I just said, "OK, thanks," and left to go home.

My husband had to leave town for a few days the following week, and we both tentatively thought I was doing better. The hangover from the incident was a fuzzy, slightly nauseous feeling, so my parents came down to stay. Within two days, we were back at the hospital, I was down again, and my parents were beside themselves.

The cycle of blinding headaches continued all that summer. After seeing a *lot* of doctors, the only diagnosis they could come to was a cycle of migraines, triggered by the change in my environment and dehydration.

In the meantime, I'd developed sinus issues and what the doctors called allergies, something I'd never had before. Allergy pills and a nasal spray were prescribed. I was also given a migraine pill that never seemed to work.

Over the next few years, the migraines continued and so did the low-level fear. "What if I get a migraine?" was always in my mind, lurking like a monster in the closet. I developed a fear of travel and was hesitant to accept invitations. I did my best, but I know I disappointed many hosts with last-minute cancelations.

We decided we wanted to have a baby. I got pregnant within six months, and I sadly remember the joy of having a baby in my belly, only to lose him at fourteen weeks. We were desolate, heartbroken, and determined. We turned to IVF and immediately conceived again, to lose the baby a week after seeing a heartbeat. It was another boy.

Something in me woke up. I was determined to make having a baby a reality. We moved on to using donor eggs. It seemed my body didn't want to carry anyone else's eggs, either. No medical professional could ever explain the losses. In one year's time, I'd been pregnant more days than not pregnant, and we still didn't have our baby.

What I did have was a lot more weight than normal, mostly from the hormone treatments. I felt like I'd aged a decade in a few short years,

and I looked it, too. I was tired all the time, I'd developed chronic sinus issues, and I had aches and pains all over. I was still in my thirties, but I felt like I was much older.

We turned to adoption the following year, and within nine months we had a bouncing, healthy baby boy from Russia. Our son had found his way to us. He was smart, savvy, and walking and talking by the time he was eleven months. He was a handful, but we felt blessed and happy beyond words.

New motherhood was challenging, and although I tried to get my health back after the miscarriages, nine months wasn't long enough. In the first year of my baby's life, I broke out in a viral rash up and down my arms and was diagnosed with mononucleosis. I was still recovering from the hormonal imbalance, and the baby's schedule left me sleep-deprived. I wasn't taking care of myself—I wasn't exercising and I wasn't paying attention to my food.

I kept going, renovating our newly acquired historic home and taking care of my baby son. By this time, I'd also stepped in to manage my husband's business, and it seemed I was needed on all three fronts, all the time. Over the next few years, I struggled with my weight, trying every diet known to man—or woman. I did protein fasts and lost seventeen pounds in a month, only to gain it back and screw up my metabolism in the process. I signed up for Weight Watchers, Jenny, and other programs; I bought every book on dieting the moment it came out. Up, down, up, down, until I finally gave up. I was worn out. I remember thinking, as I ate my son's mac and cheese, maybe this is just the way it is once you have kids. I tried to stop worrying about it.

I continued to get sick, often, and my sinuses were a constant problem. I'd developed pain points—the tender-to-the-touch points on the body that are a sign of fibromyalgia, which basically means unexplained muscle pain. It wasn't horrible, but it was always there.

"What's happening to me?" I wondered. I was in a doctor's office at least once a month. One morning, I woke with purple bruises on the inside of my finger joints. That's strange, I thought, I haven't done anything to bruise myself. My doctor took one look and said, "Rheumatoid arthritis."

The year my son turned four, I had seven sinus infections. We were forced to count them because it seemed to me that I was living on antibiotics, and my next step was surgery. Antibiotics had become my "feel good" drug, keeping the infections at bay and giving me a week or two of energy at a time. Once off the drug, I would go down again within three weeks. I'd begin to feel tired and groggy, and get frequent headaches. I had trouble getting out of bed, and I was taking antidepressants and struggling with feelings of hopelessness.

One evening, after rallying myself out of a two-week sinus infection and a migraine, I attended a lecture at a friend's home. She asked how I was doing, and hearing that this was my first night out in weeks, she looked me in the eye and said, "Have you considered that your immunity is seriously compromised? Could your diet have anything to do with all this endless illness?" Something about that shook me to my core. What could happen when your immunity is compromised? The roster of ailments and diagnoses ran through my mind that night. Infertility, allergies, migraines, fibromyalgia, rheumatoid arthritis, depression, weight gain, mononucleosis, chronic sinus infections, hopelessness . . . fear. What would be next?

The next day I decided to seek alternative help. Before my marriage, I'd managed to be pretty healthy despite all the long hours, extensive travel, and stress. I always said it was because I was something of a self-taught student of nutrition. I ate a healthy diet even while I was wining and dining—or being wined and dined—as part of my job.

Through a fog of sinus headaches and migraines, I called the nutritionist my friend had recommended. I was sick and tired of being sick and tired. I realized that carrying an extra 40 pounds or more was having an effect on everything. Based on her recommendations, I joined a CSA (community supported agriculture) farm and started receiving boxes of fresh, local, seasonal veggies every week. I started cooking every day, and vegetables became my friend again. I ate salads at every meal (even breakfast) and I gradually started to feel better. I lost a few pounds. I started walking every day and began yoga classes.

Basically, I fell in love with healthy food again. I healed, gradually. I lost weight, gradually. I began to feel like me again, ever so slowly. The migraines gradually went away. The aches and pains went away. One day, I realized that I hadn't had a sinus infection in a year. It had been so long since I'd seen him that my doctor called to see if I was OK.

By working with a holistic nutritionist, I learned that I have some food intolerances that were contributing to my aches and pains. I eliminated those foods from my diet and started to feel even better.

Healing My Son

At the age of six, my son developed symptoms similar to those I had experienced. He had a chronic cough; the doctor diagnosed asthma. He caught every virus that passed through his school for almost a year. Then he was diagnosed with mononucleosis. That was the final straw for us both. We needed to make some changes for him as well.

After consulting with his doctor, step one was to take him off all the drugs he'd been prescribed. Step two was to take him out of school for a few months to avoid the constant exposure to germs from other kids. Step three was to eliminate dairy from his diet. I cooked healthy, organic, local food every day.

At the end of three months, we visited his doctor. The doctor drew blood and ran tests; he was impressed by how much more energetic, happy, and responsive my son now was. I told the doctor what I had been doing to improve my son's immunity. He was skeptical, but said, "He looks ready to get back to school, but I'll call you in a few days with results."

When the doctor called me, he said, "Your son's tests are perfect. Please keep him off pharmaceuticals and keep him on your home remedies. They're working."

This was my turning point. I thought: What if I hadn't taken this into my own hands? What if I had kept going down the path to being overweight, tired, and exhausted all the time? What if I'd let the doctors continue to give drugs to a young child? I stood in our farm kitchen holding a green drink, wearing my skinny jeans, and watching my son run around outside with our dogs.

The thought came to me very clearly: People need to know.

I had found my passion after all. I enrolled in nutrition school to learn all I could about how food can heal. I became a Certified Holistic Health Coach (CHHC) through the Institute for Integrative Nutrition in New York City; I then became a Certified Natural Health Professional (CNHP) through the National Association of Certified Natural Health Professionals. I discovered the power of plant-based nutrition and how crucial organic and local food is to our country and to the world. I took classes in cooking and had new culinary worlds—vegetarian, vegan, raw—open to me. I began my consulting practice as a health coach specializing in nutrition. I advocated, I blogged, I took people on farm tours, I spoke to women's groups, I went on TV, and I began effecting change in my community and beyond.

I continued to shop and cook with the seasons, and I discovered the joys of seasonal eating—the feeling of being connected to my community, to local farming, and to the weather. My family loved fresh applesauce from our old apple tree in late summer, and an abundance of squash and pumpkins in the fall. We ate hearty root vegetables with warming spices in winter, and in spring the asparagus and fresh greens felt clean and light, like the season itself.

Discover Your Nutritional Style was born. I was ready to get busy, to teach and empower other women to live their purpose, to be their best self, to achieve ageless beauty, vitality, and health from the inside out, using the healing power of food. I was ready to help them find their own Nutritional Style.

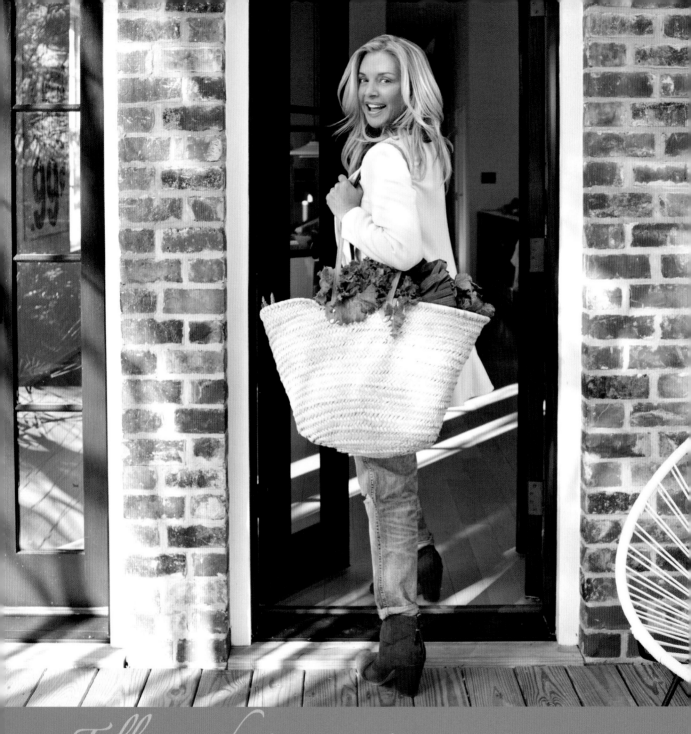

Tell me what you eat,
and I will tell you what you are.

—Jean Anthelme Brillat-Savarin, *The Physiology of Taste*, 1825

CHAPTER ONE

What's Your Nutritional Style?

The little black dress (LBD) is iconic and always in style. Think Audrey Hepburn, Jackie O, or Gwyneth Paltrow, the embodiments of effortless chic. Designers Karl Lagerfeld, Donna Karen, and Michael Kors feature LBDs regularly as the staple of any stylish woman's wardrobe. My guess is you have at least one, if not several, hanging in your closet.

The best LBDs go with anything, and can take you from a dinner party in the spring to a cocktail party in the summer to a business dinner in the fall, and still look amazing and sleek at a semi-formal holiday event.

While the little black dress is a foundation piece for any woman's wardrobe, your favorite one isn't the same as your best friend's. You adore silk, and she's comfortable in a lightweight knit. You prefer knee length, and she loves several inches higher. A high waist suits you, and her shape looks best in a straight chemise. While we all love and need our little black dresses, each of us has different preferences when it comes to this basic wardrobe item. We each choose the one that fits our personal signature look.

Once you settle on your little black dress, you adapt it as needed. You add a hot pink sweater and a colorful retro necklace with black tights and heels for the spring dinner party. Summer cocktails call for a lightweight pastel pashmina and swinging chandelier earrings to go with your suntanned legs and gold strappy sandals. You pull out a black fitted jacket for the fall business dinner, add a pop of color with a gorgeous Hermès scarf, and balance it with nude legs and nude heels, the epitome of business chic. You look drop-dead elegant at the holiday party, showing toned, bare arms, layers of pearls, and satin heels with a bow.

Not everyone has a little black dress—or feels the need for one. Maybe you're more a blue jeans and sneakers sort of person who never needs to dress up. You still make those jeans your own, because you're you, with your own unique style. Your personality comes through, no matter what you wear. And no matter what you have on, your own needs are still there.

Your Nutritional Style

Just as the little black dress is unique to you, so is your Nutritional Style. Just as the little black dress calls for different accessories throughout the seasons, your Nutritional Style must change with the seasons as well.

Your Nutritional Style is the eating style that makes you feel like the best version of you. Eating for your Nutritional Style gives you energy and allows you to live a sustainable lifestyle without causing stress and anxiety to your body or your mind.

It's not religion, and it's not scientific. It's about discovering your own best way of eating, living, and feeling great. It's the one that lets you effortlessly release excess weight and returns your natural vibrancy and glow from the inside out. Just like choosing the clothes that make you feel your best, it's about finding the Nutritional Style that works best for you.

Think of your food and nutrition as unique to you, and not as a way to fit into someone else's plan or ideal. You're not meant to live life going from diet to diet that you're either on or off, and you don't want to feel good or bad about yourself based on whether or not you stuck to a diet someone else created.

Here's the best part. Your style can, and should, evolve over time; and it can, and should, change and adapt with the seasons.

The Healthy Omnivore

An omnivore is someone who eats all kinds of foods, including both animal and plant foods. I'm using the term *Healthy Omnivore* here, not regular ol' *omnivore,* because anyone working with me is going to be the healthiest version of an omnivore possible. Animal protein includes red meat, pork, chicken and poultry, fish and all seafood, eggs, and dairy foods, including milk, butter, and cheese.

As a Healthy Omnivore, you eat lots of fresh vegetables, fruits, and an assortment of plant-based proteins, such as beans, nuts, seeds, and whole grains. You've learned to eat the right amount of animal protein, an amount that won't weigh you down or clog your digestion.

The main way omnivores get into dietary trouble is by taking this Nutritional Style too far. When you rely too heavily on animal

> Eating for your Nutritional Style gives you energy and allows you to live a sustainable lifestyle without causing stress and anxiety to your body or your mind.

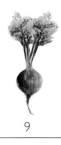

proteins, consuming them several times a day, it can lead to sluggish digestion, constipation, lack of vitality, dull skin, and weight gain in the short term. Significant health issues, such as heart disease and even cancer, could show up in the long run. Unhealthy omnivores usually indulge too frequently in processed foods, such as pizza, breads and baked goods, and low-quality snacks and sweets. These foods dull your taste for fresh ingredients and whole foods; they crowd out more nutritious foods from your diet.

If, as you read this, you realize you're an unhealthy omnivore, let's first focus on upgrading you to Healthy Omnivore status. As your eating patterns evolve, we'll revisit your eating style season by season, while still allowing you to keep the variety of foods you love.

Don't worry. If you choose this eating style for the long haul, you're in good company. Both the Dalai Lama and Michael Pollan believe that animal protein is necessary for optimal health. We're going to make you the healthiest omnivore possible.

The Flexible Vegetarian

If you're a Flexible Vegetarian, also called a Flexitarian, you follow a vegetarian or an almost vegetarian eating style. You mostly avoid animal foods and enjoy the amazing variety of plant foods: beans, nuts, seeds, grains, vegetables, and fruits. You sometimes eat some poultry or fish, and also enjoy moderate amounts of eggs and dairy foods.

I'm not using the label *vegetarian*, because your Nutritional Style isn't about rules and never eating animal foods. Many of my clients come to me already enjoying this particular eating style. They're vegetarian, except for when they're not. They don't feel guilty if they crave an egg once in a while, or if they enjoy a piece of fish while out to dinner. It's just food, and if their diet is 90 percent vegetarian, they're OK with that. Your Nutritional Style is about the style of eating that you love and that makes you feel your absolute best. It's not about forbidden foods.

The downside to the standard vegetarian diet is that people employing this style often rely too heavily on processed carbs. Many people "fail" on a vegetarian diet because they forget about the vegetable part of the word; instead, they load up on sugary carbohydrates

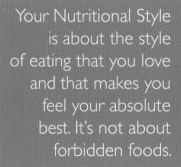

Your Nutritional Style is about the style of eating that you love and that makes you feel your absolute best. It's not about forbidden foods.

Your Nutritional Style is the style of eating that nourishes and satisfies you completely, not just because you look your best when you eat that way, but because you feel it, too. It's the style of eating that banishes cravings, feeds your body well, and allows you to live life with joy, ease, and grace. It's the style that fits well with the rest of your life and enhances it.

So what's your Nutritional Style? Let's figure that out together.

Take the quiz below and tally up your answers. When deciding which answer to give, please pick the one that's closest to your usual eating habits. Or think of it this way: If you were eating out and had to choose from the three options, which would it be?

You'll probably find you fit naturally into one of three Nutritional Styles. Once you've determined what your basic Nutritional Style is, we'll begin your journey to better health with whichever style suits you *right now*. Within that style, I'll teach you to upgrade your food choices to make them the healthiest ones possible. And if later on you feel you need to adapt your food choices to a different style, you'll have the knowledge to make the shift slowly, and seasonally, in a smart and sustainable way.

No matter which style you choose, they all share one common goal: to help you attain a fabulous, vibrant, uplifting, happy-to-be-you level of health and well-being. I invite you to find that place where you feel good in your own skin and know you're doing your best to stay there.

1. What's your preferred source of protein in the food you normally eat?

    A. Animal protein: meats, fish, eggs, maybe dairy
    B. Legumes: beans and lentils
    C. Nuts, seeds, and some soy

2. An average dinner for you would be:

    A. Chicken breast, quinoa, and veggies
    B. Vegetable chili and a salad
    C. Kale noodles and fresh marinara sauce

3. Your favorite breakfast is:

    A. Bacon and eggs
    B. Oatmeal with blueberries
    C. Green juice

4. They offer wild salmon and steak filet at a party and you choose:

    A. Both, to taste each of them
    B. A small piece of salmon
    C. That fish had a mother! Pass the salad again.

5. Your BFF wants to go for ice cream, and you get to choose what kind. You go for:

    A. Full fat and delicious creamy ice cream, any flavor!
    B. Rice milk or tofu ice cream that tastes almost as good
    C. Raw organic coconut ice cream loaded with raw cacao nibs

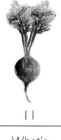

6. The soup you crave for chilly days is:

   A. Hearty chicken and vegetable, maybe add some noodles?
   B. Miso noodle soup or lentil
   C. Raw broccoli soup with tahini, warmed gently

7. How often do you eat fish?

   A. Whenever I want, as long as it's a kind I love
   B. Now and then if at all
   C. Never. Our oceans are threatened

8. How do you feel if you don't have meat, fish, or eggs for several days?

   A. I definitely miss it and want it back. Why am I doing this?
   B. I feel OK—I'm eating more legumes and grains, and I don't really miss it.
   C. Fabulous

9. What's in your omelet at the omelet bar?

   A. Ham, sausage, onions, yum
   B. Spinach, onions, a bit of cheese, and easy on the eggs
   C. Skip the eggs, please sauté all the vegetables you have.

10. You just arrived at an avant-garde cocktail party, starving, and the menu is only cheese. You go for:

    A. All of it
    B. You eat mostly the veggies and crackers, because you know you're intolerant of dairy products.
    C. You whip out a raw bar from your handbag and nibble away.

11. You just ate a big, gooey sugar doughnut from the corner doughnut chain. How do you feel?

    A. Really bad, but really good. Life happens.
    B. It was delicious, but now I'm feeling bloated. I'm juicing when I get home.
    C. Nauseated and unable to think or speak

12. What do you eat at a big holiday dinner?

    A. Turkey, ham, all the sides, and, of course, dessert. I love to taste everything!
    B. A few bites of turkey, all the sides, and I'll splurge on dessert. It's a holiday!
    C. I'll skip the meat, eat the sides that aren't too heavy in dairy or gluten, and load up on the
       vegetables. Dessert? There's always room for a little taste.

Scoring Your Nutritional Style Quiz
Tally up your total number of answers in each category.
   •   If you mostly answered As, you're a Healthy Omnivore.
   •   If you answered mostly Bs, you're a Flexible Vegetarian.
   •   If C was your favorite pick, you're a Modern Vegan.
What if your answers don't fall into a clear Nutritional Style? Or what if you think that style won't work
well for you? That's OK. By the time we get through this chapter, you'll know which style you are and
where you can go with it.

and dairy foods to replace the meat in their diet. A diet that has lots of cheese, deep-fried onion rings, and blueberry muffins isn't really a healthy diet, even if it doesn't include red meat. For too many vegetarians, an unbalanced diet leads to weight gain, low energy, skin problems, digestive issues, sinus problems, and more, all because they're making poor nutritional choices.

TINA From Omnivore to Flexible Vegetarian

When Tina first scheduled an appointment with me, she was an omnivore who ate meat at most meals. She believed that animal protein sustained her; without it, she felt weak. At the same time, she was having problems with bloating and constipation. She often had big energy drops in the afternoon, when she felt deeply tired and had trouble focusing on her work.

Tina's diet relied too heavily on animal protein for her calories. She figured her daily multivitamin filled in for the total absence of vegetables and fruit in her food. As we worked together, I recommended that Tina add more vegetables to her meals. We wanted to increase her intake of phytonutrients and essential vitamins and minerals, and also add some much-needed fiber.

Instead of eggs and toast for breakfast, I recommended she switch to eggs and sautéed spinach, or skip the eggs and go with warm grains.

Instead of a meat-filled sandwich each day, Tina began enjoying a salad with a small amount of animal protein a few days a week. She learned to vary her lunch by having lentil or bean soup or quinoa salad.

Instead of meat for dinner every night, Tina switched to meatless meals, starting just once a week and then adding a couple more days. She learned to make delicious stir-fries full of vegetables, using nuts or seeds to substitute for the meat. She also learned to make hearty bean stews and vegetarian chili. We made sure to include plenty of healthy fats—in addition to being essential to good health, the fats helped Tina feel satisfied by her food and helped sustain her energy throughout the day. Her afternoon energy lags became less severe.

Gradually, we added more and more plant foods. We began exploring protein smoothies, too. As we did, Tina's taste buds began to change. She stopped craving meat at each meal and felt satiated by all of the flavorful, fiber-rich foods she was now eating.

After about three months of gradual changes, Tina mentioned that she hadn't had meat in almost two weeks. When I asked her why, she said she'd just lost her taste for it. She also said she felt her thinking was clearer and she had more energy since she stopped eating meat. Her afternoon energy lags were gone— she was now feeling highly productive all day long.

I hadn't encouraged Tina to give up meat completely—all I did was suggest cutting back and substituting healthier choices. Likewise, Tina hadn't consciously set out to remove meat from her diet. She realized, however, that she clearly felt better and looked better now that she wasn't eating meat. She had, without really trying, found the Nutritional Style that worked for her: Flexible Vegetarian.

It's been a few years now, and Tina continues her Flexible Vegetarian Nutritional Style. She eats mostly plant-based foods, along with moderate amounts of dairy products and eggs. She eats fish now and then, and meat only rarely. She continues to feel and look great!

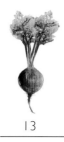

When vegetarians find their supposedly healthy diet isn't working for them, they throw up their hands, claim their hair is thinning, and say their doctor tells them to go home and eat meat. They tell themselves that they just aren't supposed to be vegetarian.

In reality, they never approached this eating style in a healthy, well-informed fashion. It's very easy to be an unhealthy vegetarian, but it's just as easy to be a super-healthy one. Flexibility is the key.

If you're a Flexible Vegetarian, you allow yourself the occasional serving of meat, poultry, fish, eggs, and dairy products, because you're aware of your body and know when it is calling for some extra protein and dietary fat. You add generous amounts of greens, vegetables, fruits, and raw foods to your diet to keep your mood balanced and your energy levels high. Most important, you eat this way because you love the taste and variety of wonderful plant-based foods. All over the world, meatless dishes are the basis of richly flavored, highly nutritious ethnic cuisines. With so many food traditions to draw on, a Flexible Vegetarian is never bored by her food!

The Modern Vegan

The fundamental principle of veganism is avoiding all animal foods—even honey, because it's made by bees—and eating only plant-based foods. Many vegans choose this path for ethical reasons: They wish to avoid harming other living things, and they wish to have a minimal impact on the environment. But being a vegan isn't a form of penance—it doesn't mean eating nothing but brown rice and steamed kale. If you're a Modern Vegan, your Nutritional Style is full of vegetables, fruits, grains, and plant-based protein sources, like dark greens, beans, nuts, and seeds. Many Modern Vegans also choose to eat mostly raw foods. If you have a good understanding of both nutrition and your own body, being a Modern Vegan can be a perfectly healthy lifestyle.

I work with many Modern Vegans in my consulting practice. The key to success for them is to be flexible in what they eat. It's OK for a Modern Vegan to indulge an occasional craving for raw sheep's milk cheese or local honey. It's OK to cut back on raw foods if your body is craving the warmth and easier digestibility of cooked foods.

It's also OK to bend a bit, especially when you're away from your own kitchen. One of my Modern Vegan clients needs to attend business luncheons a few times a month. If it's a buffet, great—there's always plenty of salad and veggies and usually a meatless choice or two. If it's a sit-down meal and there's a vegetarian option, she asks for it. If there's no vegetarian choice, and the waiter can accommodate her

KAREN To Vegan and Back

My client Karen grew up in a family that ate the Standard American Diet. Lots of boxed cereals and sugary snacks, plenty of microwaved foods, and always meat for dinner.

As an adult, Karen became more aware of what she was eating, but it took becoming a mother to decide she really needed to clean up her diet. Unfortunately, Karen didn't have a good idea of where to start. After listening to some of the moms in her children's playgroup, she decided to make a radical change in her own diet and become a vegan. She abruptly gave up all animal foods and took up juicing. At first, Karen felt amazing. She had energy to spare, enjoying huge amounts of greens and vegetables, beans, grains, nuts, and seeds. She lost weight, too. For about a year, she was happy. Then she began to crave what she was feeding her family.

She began to sneak bites of her kid's organic hot-dogs. She found herself picking at the roasted chicken in the kitchen so her husband wouldn't question her choices. She was frustrated and hungry all the time, trying hard to make her new vegan lifestyle work. She believed that being a vegan was the best choice for her (after all, the other moms seemed so happy), but her body was rebelling.

It was at this confusing time that Karen came to see me. Her head wanted one thing, but her body fought her and wanted something else. Karen was losing energy and craving food all the time. She felt like she was never satisfied by her meals, which led to frightening episodes of binge eating. On top of her out-of-control behavior, she could see that her hair was lackluster and thinning. Karen was worried.

She proudly told me she was a vegan. When she described her ideal eating day, I was confused as to why she'd called. Then she told me the true story: her diet and mind were all over the place, and she no longer knew what to do.

I knew what Karen was going through because I'd been there myself. I recommended that she let go of the dogma, the all-or-nothing attitude about her food. Her goal before our next session was to add in a serving of organic animal protein of some kind a few times that coming week, without guilt. She needed to listen to her body and eat what it told her she was craving.

Karen went for it, and within a week she was feeling like a new person. Her agitation was gone; she was calmer and stronger. She felt like working out again, and she even lost the anxious feeling that each meal would bring. She hadn't binged once that week.

We worked together for three months, and came up with many vegan and animal protein meals that worked for her because they gave her the protein and dietary fat she needed. Karen learned how to change her eating pattern seasonally and handle occasional periods of high stress. She's ditched the stigma she used to attach to eating animal protein, in favor of her own physical and mental health.

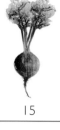

request for more broccoli and no chicken, that's fine. If not, she quietly does the best she can with whatever is put in front of her. She'll often eat—and enjoy—the animal-based main course. Remember, it's food, not religion.

If you're eating in a healthy Modern Vegan style, you're aware of how your body reacts to your food and you have a strong interest in nutrition. The downside to the vegan eating style comes if you become too dogmatic about food and diet, jumping on each new diet trend and superfood, and obsessing over your own nutrition. This can lead to ignoring signs that your body may not agree with your latest diet plan. Most Modern Vegans need a little bit of leeway, and I'm giving you the freedom to listen to your body and let go of the strict rules. (Check out chapter two for more on the importance of flexibility in your approach to food.)

Discovering Your Nutritional Style

As you can see from the quiz, discovering your Nutritional Style isn't complicated, but it is personal. What works for someone else might not be right for you. I'm pretty certain, for example, that the celebrity diet you read about at the salon while waiting for your stylist isn't going to be the best approach for you.

What is right for you could be as simple as tweaking a few things in your diet, or it might mean a bigger shift in what you eat. No matter what, the goal of finding your Nutritional Style is to make you feel beautiful and energized.

Health and beauty come from being comfortable and happy in your body, having high energy, and a love and passion for life, and knowing that you look and feel the absolute best you can.

What Are You Really Eating?

If you're like most of the women I consult with, you believe, for the most part, that you eat in a healthy way. You have a sense that you could do better, but compared to your assistant, friend, or sister, you're a health nut. She orders a greasy burger at lunch and you have a salad. While your colleagues at work are raiding the vending

I'm giving you the freedom to listen to your body and let go of the strict rules.

machines, you're enjoying healthier snacks, such as nuts or fruit. Good for you! But what about the rest of the time? Not so much.

Chances are you're eating whatever's within reach. More often than not, you ignore what you know and rationalize that "everybody else eats that way, so why not me?" You've paid the price for too long. It's time to stop. Wake up and greet the day like Mary freakin' Tyler Moore; toss that hat into the air and turn the world on with your smile. You can. Let me show you how.

You're a busy person. Most of the time, you eat what's handy— a frozen meal tossed in the microwave, last night's party leftovers, take-out from the deli near the office, or whatever the meeting coordinator is serving that day. You justify it to yourself by saying, it's here, it's easy, I'm starving, and I'll get back to eating healthily tomorrow.

When you do cook for yourself, you nibble on a favorite cheese with some crackers and pour a glass of wine to go with it. Before you know it, you've eaten several servings of the cheese and had a second glass of wine. If you do happen to become conscious of your snacking, you wonder, "Can anyone really cook a meal without appetizers and a glass of wine?" And for another day, you give up on healthy eating and decide to start again tomorrow.

The next day, you grab a candy from the bowl at the receptionist's desk, because it's there, and how bad can one little piece be? Ten luscious, high-fructose candies later, you're filled with regret and a sense of failure. "How many chocolate pieces did I just eat?" you wonder, counting the wrappers in the wastebasket. "S*#t," you murmur, and vow to eat only lettuce for lunch.

Every few weeks, you resolve to do better for your health and, let's face it, your looks. You know you could feel better, and you've read enough nutrition articles to realize you could make better choices, you just have no idea where to start or what to believe. There's so much contradictory information out there, and every day you read or hear something different. The *Today Show* brings on an expert who says eat goji berries, and the latest guest on *Good Morning America* swears by blueberries. The next day, Dr. Oz recommends a different berry that you've never heard of. Are you supposed to worry about your antioxidants that much? It makes you want to just give up and eat at the nearest fast food place.

> The best way to learn what suits you . . . is to learn to listen to your own body wisdom. You have unique nutritional needs that suit your internal make up and your lifestyle.

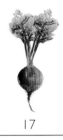

Plus, the extra weight you're carrying drives you crazy. Those extra 10 or even 20 pounds are exhausting. Your energy lags, and none of your favorite clothes fit. You've done several diets with mixed results, and while you've lost some pounds, you couldn't wait for the diet to end. Who wants to live on processed packets of powdered food that you mix with water? How healthy can it be to eat frozen meal after frozen meal? And how badly will you feel when the diet ends and, despite your effort and discipline, you put all that weight back on and more? You've had it.

Allergies, migraines, low energy, mood swings, and many other common health problems are closely linked to nutrition. Going to the doctor and collecting a medicine cabinet full of pills and sprays has helped the symptoms, but not the cause.

Let me guess. Not one of those doctors has ever asked you what you eat, have they?

After years of trying to improve your health through nutrition, you still haven't found the winning formula. All those diets and books and supplements have proven only one thing—that nothing seems to work, and you have no clue what to do about it.

With shelves of vitamin pills, and a cabinet full of expensive powders and teas, you've spent hundreds of dollars on the next big thing for weight loss or gorgeous skin, but you take whatever potion or powder it is for five days and give up, because you hate choking down fistfuls of capsules and gross powdered drinks.

The best way to learn what suits you from a nutritional point of view is to learn to listen to your own body wisdom. You have unique nutritional needs that suit your internal make up and your lifestyle. When you meet those needs you'll feel satisfied, and may even start to feel so good you will wonder how something as simple as food could make such a profound, important, and positive difference in your life.

Adapting Your Nutritional Style

Several years ago my diet consisted of almost entirely raw, vegan food. I adapted to this style of eating gradually, over a few years, and it was working for me. At my lowest weight, and with my energy sky high, I was productive and blissfully happy. I was certain I'd found a nutritional remedy I could follow for the rest of my life.

I delved into raw and vegan cookbooks, learned to prepare my food in creative and nutritious ways, got certified as a raw chef, and incorporated superfoods, nuts, seeds, smoothies, and juicing into my day. My health improved to the point where I couldn't remember the last time I'd gotten sick. It was a wonderful, healthful time.

I continued on this path for almost two years. My skin glowed from the high levels of phytonutrients, and my hair and nails grew stronger than ever before from the plant-based protein sources that my body preferred.

Then I began to sense new changes in my body—not so welcome ones this time. I began to lose circulation in my fingers throughout the day; they would turn white on one hand, sometimes both. I felt cold and was unable to get warm as winter approached.

When I first experienced these symptoms, I denied they were the result of my diet. Convinced it was happening because of unusually cold weather, I dressed in layers and turned up the heat in the house. I wore sweaters, drank a lot of tea, and continued to believe that nutritionally speaking, this was the right path. I continued to create raw food masterpieces in my kitchen while what I really craved was a big bowl of warm stew or soup.

I was cold, all the time. Despite the season, I couldn't recall ever experiencing such a chill. I didn't know it yet, but my body had begun to rebel.

As my cravings became stronger, I began to steal bigger and bigger bites of my son's dinner, and it was then that I realized that this behavior was crazy. To force myself to eat one way while my body was crying out for something else was unhealthy. It wasn't what I wanted to bring into my business and my family.

Despite my awareness of changes in my body, I felt as if I'd failed, that somehow I should have been able to make it through the winter eating a strictly vegan, raw diet. But I had to acknowledge it was taxing my system, and my diet had become unsustainable. I needed to make changes.

I began eating more steamed and roasted vegetables, stir-fried entrees, thick soups, and quinoa stews. I still ate salads loaded with superfoods and drank cacao smoothies and green juices, but the more complicated raw food preparations fell away for the time being. A new, warming, seasonal menu was nurturing and gratifying. It enabled my body to handle the cold climate.

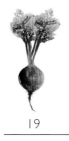

That spring and summer, my body naturally wanted to return to eating raw foods. As the warm spring air blew across our farm in northern Virginia, I added more and more fresh, local raw foods. As the summer heat soared, I craved the cooling crunch of raw vegetables and fruits, but I wasn't trying to consume only raw foods anymore—I was listening to what my body was asking for. And as the heat of the summer that year gave way to cooler nights of early fall, I was drawn again toward warm soups, roasted root vegetables, and the occasional serving of animal protein.

I'm sharing my story because, whatever your Nutritional Style, it's more important to listen to your body than it is to stick to a set of rules. Many people, especially women, seek to adopt a new strict diet or way of eating that someone else dictates. I've given up on that. I no longer follow anyone else's rules. I've learned to accept what my body wants and needs and change my eating habits accordingly around the year.

Is Your Nutritional Style Right for You?

The Nutritional Style quiz gave you a good idea of your basic approach to food, what you like, and what works best for you. But it's possible you're forcing yourself into a style that actually isn't best for you. Let's take a good, honest look at your health right now, and notice any undesirable symptoms you might be experiencing.

Are you holding onto weight, even though you're not overeating? Are you suffering from chronic headaches, sinus congestion, or frequent colds? Do you have unexplained pain, bloating, or discomfort in your stomach or gastrointestinal tract after eating? Are you frequently constipated, or do you get diarrhea, or do you alternate between the two? Are you tired, achy, maybe depressed? Do you feel exhausted or get sick often?

What about your appearance? Is your hair thinning? Is your skin itchy, or scaly, or red? Are you still getting pimples or acne? Is your skin dry and prematurely wrinkled? Are you too thin, or are you carrying a pooch of fat around the middle?

These are all signs of an imbalance in your diet caused by your day-to-day eating patterns. Something in your nutritional habits isn't working, and it's time to make a change. Based on my experience, five key factors are universal when assessing your Nutritional Style.

> To force myself to eat one way while my body was crying out for something else was unhealthy.

Begin with where you are

The first step in figuring out your Nutritional Style is to get clear on where you are now. What do you eat most of the time? How much animal protein do you consume? Do you eat beans and grains, or is your diet based on seeds, nuts, and raw plants? Are you eating so much salad that you're not getting enough calories? Are you a heavy consumer of sugar or dairy products? (I'll talk more about these in chapter three.)

Begin by first establishing what and how you eat on a normal day. Write it down, including all the snacks, and be honest with yourself. Are you getting a good range of varied foods? Is there room for improvement?

Choose what you want

Once you've acknowledged where you are, decide if you want to move toward a new style of eating. Finding your Nutritional Style is about making your own choices. It's not necessarily about eating what's in front of you, served to you at a business dinner or by a well-meaning family member. No matter what others around you say or do, what you eat is up to you and what you want.

Your Nutritional Style doesn't have to be restrictive or confining. It should give you freedom to investigate how various foods affect your body, your energy, and your moods, and make necessary changes based on your findings. Be open to some experimentation. Maybe you love beans, lentil soups, and brown rice, and you want to try a Flexible Vegetarian diet, but you're scared you'll faint or get headaches from hunger if you don't eat meat once a day. Well, if you want to eat mostly vegetables and grains and some meat, why not? It's your choice. You get to make the rules. Finding your Nutritional Style means creating the diet that suits you, and only you.

Be ready to change and adapt

You learned from my personal story that my Nutritional Style not only evolved, but that it continues to evolve over time. I had to adapt my Nutritional Style to account for colder weather, or else. You may well want and need different foods at different times too. The most common adaptation is with the seasons, but sometimes other situations also demand adapting—recovering from a serious illness, for

> You need to learn to trust yourself, and to make the connection between the foods you eat and how you feel.

example, or trying to get pregnant. Listen to your body and, if you have a health issue, talk to a knowledgeable nutrition expert.

We're naturally inclined to eat in a way that corresponds to the time of year—our instinct is rooted in millennia of seasonal cellular programming. We crave warming foods in the fall and winter and cleansing, cooler foods in spring and summer. This book contains a chapter about each season, and how adapting to the seasons can enhance your Nutritional Style and your life.

Your Nutritional Style can also evolve over time. For example, your diet now may include a lot of meat, but after implementing some healthy upgrades and ditching those dangerous liaisons I'll talk about in chapter three, you may find you want less and less meat and are drawn to more plant-based meals. Your style will shift as you begin to let go of foods that your body doesn't like any more; you'll start to crave and reach for healthier alternatives. You'll probably find that simple changes—swapping a snack of cheese and crackers for a crispy apple, for instance—can make a surprisingly big difference.

Part of adapting your eating style will be to discover any lurking food intolerances. In chapter four, I'll take you through a semiannual seasonal cleanse plan that will allow you to figure out the source of your symptoms, isolate the foods that cause problems, and work on reducing or eradicating irritating foods from your eating style.

Tune in to your body

Truly listening to your body is the most challenging part of finding your Nutritional Style. You will learn to trust yourself, and to make the connection between the foods you eat and how you feel.

Learning to tune in to signs of imbalance is an integral part of figuring out your Nutritional Style. Often the messages indicate an intolerance or sensitivity to one or more inflammatory food groups. Gluten, sugar, and dairy are the big three offenders to look at first, and I'll help you figure out which of those bad boys is your nemesis.

You may not want to hear the message your body is sending because you love the Good Humor guy more than your boyfriend. You'd duel at sundown for a slice of your mother's lasagna, and the corner bakery's scones are worth a $15 cab ride. It's easier and more delicious to ignore the signs. I get it—that splash of vanilla cream in your coffee is so comforting it can't possibly be causing chronic sinus issues, can it? Sorry, Charlie.

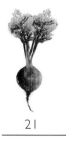

Finding your Nutritional Style is about tuning in to your body, listening to what it's saying, believing that food *is* that powerful, and making changes to correct what's not working for you at this time. Sadly, most people wait until they are faced with a life-threatening health issue before they are willing to radically change any eating patterns. (I'll talk a lot about that in chapter five, Healing in Style.) You don't need to wait until circumstances become dire to begin making changes. You're already getting signals that you need to improve your nutrition. Listen to the signs and messages that your body's sending—in chronic ailments, weight you can't lose, bad skin, and low energy.

Get smart and stand up for your own health. Make the connection between what's on your plate and health issues. See the difference in the mirror, on the scale, and maybe even in your blood test results. Feel it in your joints, in your digestion, and in your energy levels.

Add in the good and ditch the Bad Boys

No matter what your Nutritional Style is now, and regardless of where your diet is headed this year, or next, there are some truths that are self-evident. Adding in more fresh, seasonal, organic vegetables is paramount and will benefit you, no matter what else you eat. If you do just one thing for your health today, have a serving of vegetables instead of those fries or that dinner roll. As a juice or smoothie, sautéed, grilled, mashed or roasted, stir-fried, slow-cooked, or julienned, raw or steamed, they're all good.

Simple? Yes. Heard it before? Of course.

But unless you accept that your body needs nutrients that you can only get from whole foods, not a multivitamin pill, and unless you incorporate this simple act and begin to do this now, all of the benefits of the other changes you're about to make will be minimized.

No pill or supplement can give you the complex synergy of nutrients that whole plants can. Adding more vegetables into your diet, however you do it, will make a huge difference in your overall appearance and vitality.

Throughout this book, I'll talk about fun, easy, delicious ways to eat lots of veggies without feeling like you've turned into a rabbit, walking around with nothing but carrot sticks and chomping on celery all day. You'll learn how to find what's fresh and in season, the

> We all have other issues. If you begin with your food, and care about what you put into your mouth, the rest of your life does get easier.

importance of variety, and the benefits of fresh, whole foods packed with phytonutrients, year-round. You may even learn to love it. Hop on the veggie wagon with me today! It's a fun ride that'll change your life.

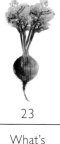

A Better Life

A better life isn't all about the food, but if we begin with our food, the rest gets easier.

When I work with my clients to find their Nutritional Style, I always start with, "Let's talk about food." It's not *all* about the food, and there are many other factors that play into our health and well-being: stress, anxiety, peer pressure, lack of time, illness, depression, allergies, bad marriages, bad relationships, toxic environments—you can name your stressor here. We all have other issues. If you begin with your food, and care about what you put into your mouth, the rest of your life does get easier.

Play with me for a minute: As your diet changes and you discover the foods that feed you well, and those that don't, you gain more energy and become open to moving more. All of a sudden, that yoga class or daily half-hour walk isn't an impossible task. After two weeks of moving, and getting your newly discovered muscles to yoga class or out for brisk walk, you begin to have more mental clarity. That project you've been postponing for months is now getting done, ten times easier than you thought. Boom!

You begin to cook at home more, and your family loves it. You're feeling good about yourself, your body feels lighter and more "yours," and you're loving your new level of productivity. Romance seems hot again, and now, everybody is *ecstatic*. Life is as it should be, delicious.

Impossible? Not your story? Maybe not exactly, so come up with your own dream. But dream big, because when you begin to eat better and feel better, and clear away the foggy brain and tired body, all things become possible.

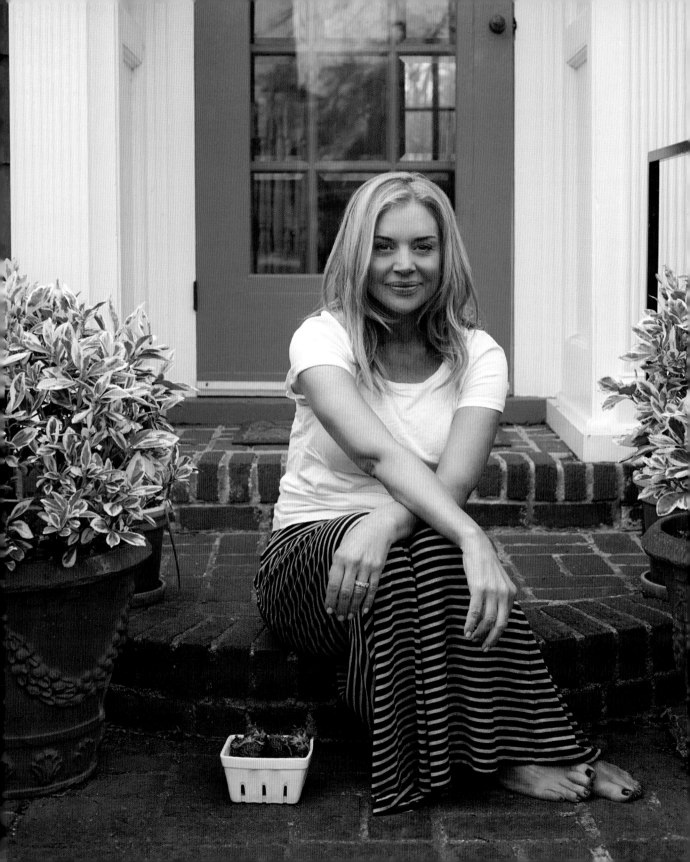

CHAPTER TWO

It's Food, Not Religion

I know you're exposed to a lot of diet hype. You might hear about a popular actress who's become a vegan, and you're sure that your skin will glow like hers if you never consume another animal product. Or you clicked on one of those Web ads that promises one weird food trick to lose a pound a week effortlessly, and now you're out a bunch of money on worthless supplements. Your best friend has given up all grains and lost 10 pounds in a month, and with a high school reunion coming up, you want to as well. Maybe that new diet book encourages you to do a five-day juice fast, and even though it's January and you live in a frigid climate, you think that sounds fabulous and fun. That 90-day liquid diet worked really well, until it was time to reenter the world of whole foods. Then you gained all the weight back, plus ten more pounds.

No matter what the hot new plan is, and no matter how healthy it seems, no regimen is going to work for everyone all of the time. In fact, any regimen that's unrelated to the way we eat in the real world and the foods that make you feel best is going to fail in the end.

Food isn't meant to be a contest with yourself—or anyone else. You won't win a prize by doing the longest juice fast, or drinking lemon and cayenne pepper for days, or losing ten pounds in a week only to gain it all back the following month. It's easy to be influenced by those around you, and the most well-meaning friends might unintentionally make you feel like you're missing out or doing something wrong. You are unique, evolving all the time, and life is in a constant state of change. What works for someone else—and did it really work?—may not work for you, or might even be harmful.

Tell me what you want to be, and I will tell you what to eat.

Discover Your Nutritional Style

The idea that your diet can be handed to you wrapped in a bow with written directions and color photos may *seem* appealing, but the reality is that no one can figure this out for you but you. The best news is that you don't want anyone else to dictate what you eat any more than you want your mother to choose your bras, or your boss to tell you how to cut your hair.

When it comes to food, you want the freedom and the power to make your own choices. I used to bury my peas in my mashed potatoes when I was a kid, so I wouldn't have to eat them. It was bad enough having the grown-ups make me eat things when I was a kid; having someone tell me as an adult what to eat would feel absurd.

One of the main reasons diets fail is *because* they're too restrictive. No one knows your body like you do. No one else knows what you love to eat, and no one can tell you what your body is going to need next week, never mind months from now.

MOTHERS AND CHILDREN Obsessed with Weight

I wish I had a bag of chia seeds for every woman I've met who has a weight problem based on something her mother said or did to her when she was young. Many of my clients had mothers who were obsessed with their own food issues and maintaining their weight. They were unable to avoid sharing their obsession with their daughters.

I've listened to beautiful and successful adult women break down in tears as they recalled specific times when their mothers' behavior toward food made them anxious or obsessive about their own food.

Times when their mothers projected their own behavior onto their daughters, telling them they needed to lose just a tiny bit, so they could look better in clothes. Or gave them smaller portions than their brothers at dinner, because us girls need to watch our weight, right? Or took them shopping at the store that sells clothes for bigger girls, because you won't look good in normal teenage clothes, sweetie, and then out

to a favorite lunch spot for salad, only.

Yes, it happens. Sadly, I'm sure those mothers meant well and loved their daughters dearly. And yet, we are hypersensitive to our mothers' suggestions. We identify with their choices, and we often choose to either model them or rebel.

For those mothers, food and weight had become obsessive and were tied to distorted emotions of self-acceptance, love, hate, success, and failure. As the daughters of these women struggle with their own identities, they often develop serious issues around eating. At worst, they develop eating disorders such as anorexia or bulimia that can be serious and even life-threatening. While I can help someone learn to eat more healthfully and sensibly, or help someone lose weight in a safe way, eating disorders are beyond my scope. When a client comes to me for help with an eating disorder, or if I feel her health or nutritional concerns are really an unrecognized eating disorder, I immediately refer her to an expert therapist.

Clients often come to me after following detailed diets that laid out every food to the last half ounce. They want me to help them stick to the diet. I tell them, "It's food, not religion. Let's not talk about guilt and sticking to impossible diets. Let's talk instead about what you like to eat and what makes you feel happy and healthy. Let's figure out your Nutritional Style and go from there." Then we throw out their food diaries and toss the powdery meal packets.

Eat What You Love, Love What You Eat

Enjoying your food is a beautiful, healthful practice. Sadly, it's something we've stopped valuing in our society. Too often we see food as the enemy, something to be wrestled with instead of embraced. Or we see food as a prescription, not sustenance. We eat something we don't like because it's supposed to be "good" for us, or avoid something we love because it's "bad" for us, or follow a diet that's supposed to prevent aging or illness. This sort of white-knuckle nutrition can't be kept up for long—it's far too scary and limiting. Even worse, we see food as a penance. We go on restrictive diets to make up for over-indulging during the holidays or on our birthday. The diet never lasts, of course, and we feel guilty and ashamed for giving up on it.

My goal in this book is to help you regain pleasure in eating by helping you choose the foods you like best and that like you best in return. Learning which foods make you feel good is empowering; you're not choosing foods based on what you can't have, you're choosing based on what makes you feel best and what you love. As we move through the seasons in this book, I invite you to connect with not only what your body needs, but also with what it wants. Not a junk food kind of want, but a *true* want. With practice, you can learn to listen to your cravings and the signals your body sends and develop a relationship of trust with your body.

By making these choices and learning what your body likes best, you can avoid the sense of failure that comes from "going off" a diet. You'll avoid the guilt that comes with the inevitable rebellion and rebound, when you find yourself chin-deep in a pint of Ben & Jerry's. And you'll avoid the temptation to turn every mouthful into an internal battle that leaves you feeling ashamed because you ate something that you should have avoided. When you understand your own Nutritional Style, you know that very few foods are on the strictly forbidden list. Instead, you understand that flexibility and variety in your food is essential.

Learning about the foods you eat and their effect on you may seem like more work, but that little bit of extra effort enables you to live the life you're meant to live—easy, graceful, and at a body weight that feels right for you, with glowing skin and vibrant eyes, and a smile on your beautiful face.

Let go of the nutrition dogma, and let me help you learn to listen to your body and discover your own Nutritional Style.

I'm not trying to make you a nutrition fanatic. I don't believe it's healthy to obsess over food. I don't believe in counting . . . fat grams,

ASTRID Stop Counting and Start Enjoying

Astrid came to me for help with her nutrition, wanting to improve what looked on the surface to be a stellar diet. Formerly overweight, her days were now filled with superfood smoothies, green juice, raw salads, healthy proteins, and very little sugar or inflammatory foods. After we spoke about her foods and lifestyle, I had some suggestions for Astrid, but overall I felt her diet was well-balanced and sustainable. She was happy about her body weight, and she worked out every day without fail.

As we spoke more, however, I began to sense a rigidity that concerned me. Astrid related stories about how her girlfriends' diets weren't as healthy as hers, how her husband ate too much sugar, and how her neighbors gave their kids processed snacks all the time. She talked about finding the best prices on superfoods and deciding the night before what she would eat the next day. I think the final straw for me was when she shared that she tallied her calories and the foods she'd consumed each day in a small spiral notebook she kept in her handbag.

I believed that Astrid was suffering from mild orthorexia, an overly rigid approach to eating. When I explained this to her, she told me that her approach to food was making her miserable—her life had been all about her food since she'd lost weight years ago.

I recommended that Astrid relax about writing everything down and allow herself frequent rewards and splurges. That advice wasn't what she'd expected to hear from me—she was expecting praise for her rigidity and near-obsession over food and even more rules for what to eat and not eat.

As part of her new goal to relax a bit about food, I asked Astrid to "allow" herself a treat every few days. Her goal was to enjoy, savor, and delight in whatever she was eating. The only thing I wanted her to write down in her little notebooks was how much she enjoyed her organic dark chocolate bar, or the buckwheat pasta with peanut sauce, or whatever she chose as a treat. (We stayed within healthy but delicious boundaries!)

After working with me for a couple of months, Astrid felt more relaxed about her foods. She was no longer gripping her grocery shopping cart, tight-lipped and concerned, as she marched up and down the supermarket aisles. Instead, Astrid was smiling. Releasing her nutrition rubber band to extend out for occasional treats and splurges made her happier than she had been for a long time.

sugar grams, carbohydrates, vitamin levels, or even calories for that matter. You don't want to live that way for the rest of your life, so why do it now? It's time to start eating in a sustainable, life-promoting, and forever way.

When you eat appropriately for your personal Nutritional Style, your nutrition and food habits are like a giant rubber band. Your Nutritional Style holds you firmly but flexibly in place; it expands and contracts with you. You mostly stick with the fresh, seasonal foods you know are best, but you also cut loose at Sunday morning brunch and indulge in your husband's homemade waffles with maple syrup. Whatever you choose for your occasional indulgence may not be ideal, but you enjoy it. And because you are comfortable with your Nutritional Style, you easily snap back to your regular pattern the next morning.

During other times of the year, your rubber band stretches a little farther. Maybe it's during the holidays when, like most people, you eat foods that you normally avoid or that come around only during this season. It starts on Thanksgiving, when you enjoy your mother's candied sweet potatoes with marshmallows. Without flexibility, you eat too much. The next day you feel horrible and have a stomachache; instead of feeling happy to have enjoyed your family's traditions, you head to a cocktail party, drink way too much wine, and lose control at the appetizer platter. And so it goes. With flexibility, however, you make yourself and your mother happy by eating a moderate portion, just enough to enjoy the treat but not so much to throw your Nutritional Style out the window.

Sometimes you stretch your rubber band beyond what's comfortable—you might even think it's snapped for good. Don't beat yourself up and decide that you're just destined to be sick and overweight. All it takes to get things under control again is falling back on your own Nutritional Style. You know that style—it's full of the foods that satisfy you and keep you healthy. A few days of eating your own way and your rubber band will be strong and flexible once again. You'll feel resolved to eat well most of the time and enjoy a treat now and then without guilt. Your Nutritional Style is back. You wake up feeling bright-eyed and productive because you've returned to the style of eating that makes you feel energized and light.

The importance of the rubber band perspective is that it's sustainable. It's not just about avoiding headaches, or a puffy belly the

> I don't believe it's healthy to obsess over food. I don't believe in counting . . . fat grams, sugar grams, carbohydrates, vitamin levels, or even calories for that matter.

next day. It's not about losing weight, or whether or not you "cheat" or "go off" a diet. Discovering and eating within your Nutritional Style lets you enjoy delicious, nourishing foods and drinks that will support you for the rest of your life.

JANE — Permission to Adapt and Adjust

My client Jane was a classic Modern Vegan when we met. She described herself as "pretty much vegan," which I took to mean, you're vegan, except for when you're not. She had strong vegan intentions for her food, not her entire lifestyle. She loved the idea of being a vegan and not consuming animal flesh. I get that.

Jane shared a story with me that impressed me as a sign of someone who had learned to tune in to her desires and cravings around food, in a healthy way. The week before, Jane had been traveling on business with her associates. She worked for a high-end investment firm and felt the pressures of her job; working with all men in this masculine environment was often challenging.

As she put it, they don't get my green juice–toting ways, and God forbid that any one of them eat a salad. Ever.

One night on a business trip, the colleagues decided to visit a high-end steak house. She cringed, but said nothing, certain she'd find something to eat there (we'd spent a lot of time on that). When she walked in, Jane couldn't face eating a cold salad. She felt a craving for some kind of animal protein—plus she knew her colleagues would make negative comments if that was all she ate. She felt guilty, but ordered a salmon steak.

She related the story to me the next day about how badly she felt she needed something more than greens, and how good her body felt after eating the salmon. She realized she hadn't ruined her life by eating salmon, and she felt great the next day, too. She decided, with some leeway and encouragement from me, to add the occasional piece of fish back into her diet, if that's what she was feeling the need to eat.

After a few weeks of enjoying fish a couple of times a week, Jane's energy had improved and she felt more balanced and even-keeled. By working with me, she realized that what she ate didn't have to be defined by someone else; she didn't need anyone's permission to eat what she wanted and felt she needed. Jane is still pretty much a Modern Vegan and doesn't eat animal foods often, but when she does, she's fine about it.

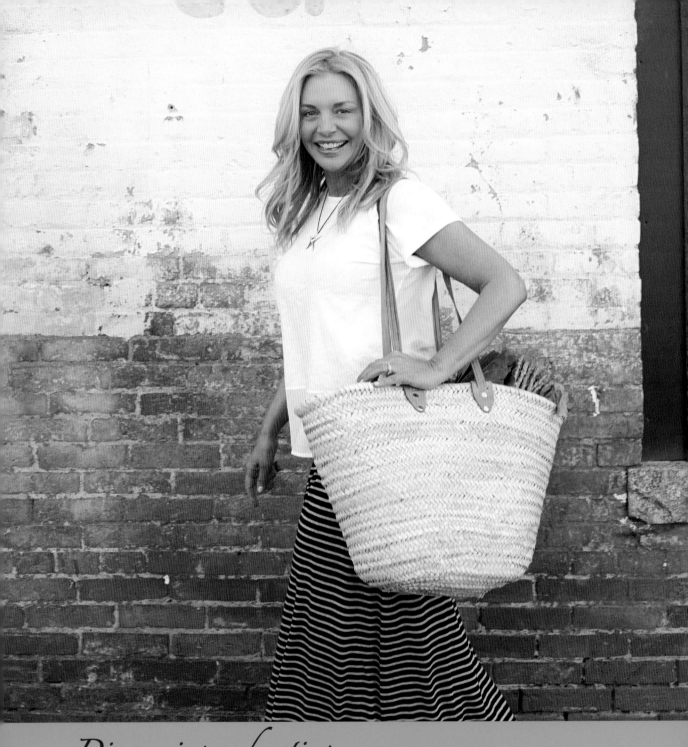

Discovering and eating within your Nutritional Style
lets you enjoy delicious, nourishing foods and drinks that will support you for the rest of your life.

CHAPTER THREE

Dangerous Liaisons

Some foods just aren't good for anyone, including you. I call them the Dangerous Liaisons, because they only mean trouble. They're toxic and potentially dangerous for your health, and I want you to avoid them wherever and however possible. I'm giving this to you straight and upfront because I want you to begin this process of getting real about your food and its effect on your body. The sooner you get that and cut these nasty boys off, the better.

Like any dangerous liaisons, some are worse than others. Some are the liaisons I call the Bad Boys: Think of Johnny Depp as the greaser gang leader in the movie *Cry-Baby*, or Jim Stark, played by real-life bad boy James Dean in *Rebel Without a Cause*, or even the dangerously sexy vampire Edward Cullen in the *Twilight* series. These guys may look enticing, but you've learned the heartache isn't worth it. It's best to stay away.

Well, it's the same with certain foods. You know they're bad for you and that if you indulge your happiness will be short-lived, but you succumb anyway. Once in a while you enjoy the sensations—the satisfaction of knowing it feels so good to be bad. It's so delicious in the moment, who cares that the next day you'll regret it? You know in your heart that a steady diet of this would make you sick and exhausted. Still, these Bad Boys wear you out, but they don't kill you.

Then there are the *really* bad guys. I call these dangerous liaisons the Serial Killers: the good-looking blind date your roommate said was antisocial and weird, or the one who hates his mother and lives in a crummy apartment with blackened windows. You'd be an idiot to date him; you know the type and you know to stay away. You're not that desperate for company, and you're not that hungry.

The tricky part is that one woman's Bad Boy could be another woman's Serial Killer. How to know? If you experience severe symptoms of food intolerance after a dangerous liaison, you've found yourself a killer. (I'll say much more about those guys later.) For now, move away from these characters. Just walk calmly in the other direction and pretend you never saw them. That's right, just keep walking.

The Bad Boys

For most of us, the Bad Boys are OK in small doses—meeting for coffee, maybe, but not dinner and a movie, and most definitely not the night. The Bad Boys tend to be gluten, dairy, processed soy foods, sugar, and, for some, caffeine.

Gluten

Gluten is a kind of protein found in the grains wheat, barley, and rye. That means gluten is found in any food made with wheat flour, including bread, cereal, pasta, baked goods, beer, and many more foods (see the chart on page 36). This Bad Boy can undermine your looks and overall health. If you turn out to be highly intolerant, eliminating gluten can change your life and rock your world.

Gluten messes with your ability to absorb nutrition in your small intestine. It can cause an immune response that damages the inner lining of the small intestine and leads to an inability to absorb nutrients well.

ISABELLE AND THOMAS   Changing a Young Life

A few years ago, Isabelle came to me to talk about her son, Thomas. At the age of five, Thomas had a lot of allergies, a constant runny nose, and frequent illness. Isabelle had taken her son to many doctors, who had put him through numerous tests and treatments, but nothing seemed to help. Her mother's intuition told Isabelle that something in Thomas's diet was the real problem, but none of the doctors were interested in following up on his nutrition.

When we talked about the family history, I learned that his grandmother had celiac disease. In fact, because celiac is often passed on genetically, Thomas had been tested for it—with negative results. As I explained to Isabelle, the test ruled out celiac disease, but it didn't rule out gluten intolerance. Isabelle agreed when I suggested removing gluten from Thomas's diet for a couple of weeks, just to see if it helped relieve his symptoms.

It's not easy to take away bread, pasta, breakfast cereal, and cookies from a five-year-old. Isabelle and I took a trip together to a nearby well-stocked health food store. We were able to find gluten-free substitutes for pretty much everything Thomas liked to eat.

I wasn't sure if Isabelle could stick with the program—Thomas was definitely strong-willed about his favorite foods. Within just a week, Thomas was so much better that Isabelle decided to extend the trial for a month. At the end of that time, Thomas was a different boy. He no longer fought chronic colds and viruses. The chronic mucus and coughs were gone. Today, he's growing tall and thriving.

Isabelle noticed that because she was sharing the foods Thomas ate, she was feeling better too! She converted her entire home to a gluten-free zone and has even gone on to persuade the local pizzeria to offer gluten-free pies.

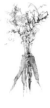

People who have celiac disease, an autoimmune condition, can't eat gluten at all. It can make them extremely ill, usually with diarrhea and abdominal pain. Celiac disease is the most severe form of gluten intolerance. It's usually diagnosed in childhood; the only treatment is lifelong avoidance of gluten-containing foods.

True celiac disease is rare, but an intolerance for gluten, ranging from mild to severe, isn't. The symptoms of gluten intolerance include diarrhea, bloating, gas, a sense of fullness, stomachache, and abdominal pain. Not all symptoms of gluten intolerance are in your digestive system, however. You might feel brain fog after eating a big bowl of pasta, or you might be irritable or depressed (too much time with Bad Boys can do that to you). A scaly, itchy skin rash known as dermatitis herpetiformis is another common sign.

Gluten intolerance used to be considered rare, but more and more research is showing that it's a lot more common than we once thought. You could have a lot of expensive blood tests to check for gluten intolerance, but there's a much simpler approach: Cut gluten out of your diet for a couple of weeks and see what happens. If you're like some of my clients, you'll be amazed at how much better you feel in just a few days. Gone are the annoying, embarrassing digestive problems that sent you scurrying out of the room.

Avoiding gluten is hard because it's everywhere. Your morning toast and cereal, your lunchtime sandwich, your doughnut or crackers in the break room, your pasta at dinner, the croutons in your salad, the cookies for dessert—they all contain gluten. In addition, gluten is often added to foods and even medications. (The chart on page 36 shows some of the surprising ways gluten can find its way into you.) So, even if you have just a mild intolerance, you could still be getting so much gluten all day long that it's seriously affecting you.

Because so many people have found that they have some degree of gluten intolerance, a whole industry of gluten-free foods has sprung up. This is a good thing—people with gluten intolerance deserve sandwiches and dessert, too—but be cautious. Sugar is a Bad Boy, and in gluten-free foods, sugar fills in for the wheat. It's like ditching the Bad Boy biker to take up with the Bad Boy meth dealer.

If you're highly intolerant, giving up gluten can change your life. You might discover that the symptoms you thought were yours to live with forever can go away just through changing your eating habits. It's not that hard.

SYMPTOMS OF GLUTEN INTOLERANCE

The symptoms of gluten intolerance can vary quite a bit, which is why it is often misdiagnosed or even ignored. The symptoms can range from diarrhea and abdominal pain to irritability to infertility.

Common Symptoms

Abdominal bloating and pain
Constipation
Diarrhea
Gas
Pale, foul-smelling, or fatty stool
Vomiting
Weight loss

Less Common Symptoms

Arthritis
Bone or joint pain
Bone loss or osteoporosis
Canker sores inside the mouth
Depression or anxiety
Fatigue
Infertility or recurrent miscarriage
Irregular menstrual periods
Irritability
Iron-deficiency anemia
Itchy skin rash
    (dermatitis herpetiformis)
Seizures
Tingling or numbness in the
    hands and feet (neuropathy)

Gluten-free grains and seeds, such as oats, quinoa, corn, brown rice, and millet, taste great and are just as nutritious, if not more so, than wheat, barley, and rye. Food manufacturers are producing better-tasting gluten-free breads, crackers, baked goods, and other foods all the time. A word of caution here: The term "gluten-free" does not necessarily mean healthy; it just means no gluten. Processed foods of any kind are Bad Boys, with or without gluten.

Avoiding gluten is a bit of a challenge. If you're only slightly sensitive, you can probably tolerate the small amounts that turn up in apparently innocent items such as ketchup and canned soup. The more intolerant you are, the more vigilant you need to be about reading food labels and questioning waiters. You'll also want

FIND THE HIDDEN GLUTEN

If you're gluten intolerant, you already know to avoid wheat, barley, and rye. Oats and oat flour don't contain gluten—in fact, oats are a common substitute in gluten-free baked goods. However, because oats often are processed using equipment that also handles other grains, buy only organic brands that state certified gluten-free on the label. In addition, some people with celiac disease or gluten sensitivity also react to oats—if you have gluten symptoms after eating oats, you might be one of them.

Gluten is also found in some nutritional supplements (vitamins, minerals, herbs, etc.) and in some prescription and nonprescription drugs. It's even in some lip balms and lipsticks!

Wheat by Other Names

Bran
Bulgur
Farina
Farro
Graham flour
Kamut
Semolina
Spelt
Triticale
Wheat germ

Dairy Products

Ice cream
Frozen dairy products (e.g., frozen yogurt)
Cheese spreads
Fruit-added yogurt (plain yogurt is usually safe)

Processed Foods

Candy bars
Chocolate
Energy bars
Hot chocolate mixes
Hot dogs
Hydrolyzed vegetable protein (read the label)
Luncheon meats
Peanut butter
Sausages
Soup: canned, mixes, bouillon cubes

Condiments

Breading and coating mixes
Drink mixes
Gravy and sauce mixes
Ketchup
Marinade mixes
Mustard
Nondairy creamers
Salad dressings
Soy sauce

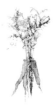

to separate your appliances, cutlery, and kitchen equipment, so you don't inadvertently contaminate gluten-free items with those that contain gluten, even in small traces.

Dairy

Dairy is the perfect Bad Boy. Delicious and highly addictive, you wish you could have it every darn day, all day, but the truth is you'd end up fat, pasty, and inflamed. I apologize in advance to all the beautiful dairy cows I've met in my lifetime—and I live in a rural area, so I've met a lot of them. I admire your production capabilities, dear cows, but giving you up has changed my life, and my son's life, forever.

In fact, the perils of milk-based foods are the main reason I wrote this book. Once I realized that many of my health problems, and those of my son, were based on eating dairy foods, our lives changed for the better. Eliminating dairy from our diets made a huge difference in our health.

Why? First of all, many people who eat dairy foods find that they stimulate mucus production. Your doctor will say that's a myth. It's true that not everyone who drinks milk or enjoys yogurt, cheese, or ice cream will produce more mucus, but many people have noted a

HAILEY A Problem with Gluten

Cutting out the gluten can really help your appearance. My client Hailey came to me with constant bloating and belly fat she just couldn't lose. She was otherwise trim, and at age 33, she felt it was too early to have that midriff stuff going on! I assured her that nobody needs that at *any age*, and we got to work. Hailey told me her mom had carried the same type of belly fat her entire adult life and had also had endless, undiagnosed digestive issues. Hailey herself had periodic flare-ups of digestive problems, especially loose bowels after meals. The problem came and went, but Hailey would just vaguely attribute it to something she ate and never tried to pin down exactly what that was. She still had good energy and was able to do her design job well, so she never thought to visit the doctor or explore the source of this uncomfortable condition.

For many of us, it's only when food intolerances begin to affect our outward appearance that we make that move to investigate further. With Hailey, a looming trip to Hawaii with her boyfriend made her decide to schedule an appointment with me. There's nothing like the prospect of being seen in a bikini to get your butt in gear! Tracking down the source of Hailey's digestive upsets and stubborn belly fat was relatively painless. We started with gluten, the most likely of her favorite Bad Boys. Hailey was very motivated to try going gluten-free for a couple of weeks. She started to lose the bloat within a week, showing that gluten truly was her problem.

distinct connection between these foods, their endless runny nose, and their allergy and sinus symptoms. The reason is the casein in milk. It turns out that a lot of people are allergic to this protein, and the allergy often shows up as increased mucus production. It can also show up as skin rashes, eczema, hives, diarrhea, cramping, bloating, and gas. Whenever a client comes to me about her mysterious rashes, we cut dairy, especially cheese, out of the diet for a couple of weeks. The rashes almost always clear up and stay away as long as casein stays out of the diet.

Because casein is digested fairly slowly, you may not make the connection between your snack of milk and cookies at 2:00 p.m. and waking up feeling horribly congested the next morning. But if you've got sinus trouble that just won't go away, or if your kid always has a chesty cough, try cutting this Bad Boy out of the diet for just a week. You'll probably notice a big difference. And something to think about: casein from milk is the stuff used in glue—it's why Elsie the Cow is on the Elmer's glue bottle.

Another reason dairy is such a Bad Boy is that while that sweet, creamy ice cream tastes great going down, it's another story once it hits your digestive system. A surprisingly large number of adults are actually lactose intolerant. They no longer produce lactase, the enzyme you need to break down and digest lactose, the sugar in milk. Most adults who can still produce lactase are of northern European ethnic heritage. The rest of us, which means the majority of people in the United States, usually lose the ability to make the enzyme sometime in late childhood or even sooner.

WENDY   Dairy Deletion

My client Wendy came to me because she had chronic mucus and frequent colds, and she was constantly visiting her doctor. Her allergy tests didn't reveal anything that made a difference. As usual, none of her doctors asked her about her diet.

I had a suspicion that dairy was the cause—it often is when mucus is an ongoing problem. Armed with recipe ideas that would please her and her family, Wendy and I went shopping for dairy-free alternatives. We replaced the milk in her morning coffee with almond milk; we found alternative snacks for string cheese and yogurt. It was fairly easy to just swap out recipes with dairy for those without. The hard part was the ice cream. Wendy was very resistant to giving up her favorite treat, but I persuaded her to try sorbets and granitas instead. Within a week, the mucus subsided, and she felt so good that she called me crying with happiness. Today Wendy remains symptom-free as long as she skips the dairy—plus she looks ten years younger.

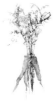

If you can't digest lactose, you know it: You quickly get gas, bloating, abdominal pain, and sometimes diarrhea. Unfortunately, milk, ice cream, yogurt, and other lactose-containing foods are very popular. They're also heavily marketed (got milk?) and are actually mandated as part of school lunches. By pushing milk and dairy products on our kids, we're doing a lot more harm than good. How many kids complain of stomachaches on school days, only to be told they're worried about that spelling test when it's really the milk they're drinking? Humans are the only mammals that continue to drink milk after they're weaned; they're also the only mammals that drink the milk of another species. Milk is for baby calves, not people.

Another big problem with dairy is that it's addictive. We all scream for ice cream; we love cheese on everything. A dairy-free life seems dull and flavorless.

But dairy is one of the first things I look for when a client tells me she can't lose those last ten or fifteen pounds. She's often eating cheese or some kind of dairy on a daily basis, and it shows. Cheese is her snack of choice before dinner, or she needs to add a splash of milk to drink her morning coffee. Been there, done that.

If you're sensitive, eating dairy can show up on your beautiful face. I've learned to recognize excessive or even daily dairy consumption as an overall puffy appearance in some people. I've seen clients who gave up dairy develop a gorgeous set of cheekbones and that toned look to their face that they always coveted, but never knew they could have. Remember, you are what you eat, and who wants to look like cheese?

For those of you who crave and need the dairy fix, there is relief. Most people with lactose intolerance can handle small amounts of dairy every now and then, especially if you have it as part of a larger meal. So yes, you can splurge on a small scoop of ice cream at your birthday dinner. You may find that dairy products with less lactose, such as yogurt and hard cheese, are OK in small amounts. Soft goat cheese and sheep cheese have a fat structure somewhat different from cow cheeses, so you may find them more digestible. You can also try lactose-free and reduced lactose milk and dairy products— these products have the lactase enzyme added to them. Milk alternatives, such as almond milk, coconut milk, and hemp milk, are good alternatives to regular milk. Over-the-counter lactase enzyme drops or tablets help some people.

CALCIUM SOURCES

The RDA for calcium is 1,000 milligrams a day for adults up to age fifty; after that, the amount goes up to 1,200 mg a day. Dairy foods are high in calcium, but as you can see from the chart, you still have plenty of other good ways to get calcium from your food. Nuts, beans, and those dark leafy greens are great sources.

Food	Amount	Calcium (mg)
Almonds	1 ounce	80
Black beans	1 cup	47
Broccoli, cooked	1/2 cup	36
Cabbage, cooked	1/2 cup	25
Chick peas	1 cup	78
Collard greens, cooked	1/2 cup	15
Kale, cooked	1/2 cup	47
Kidney beans	1 cup	50
Milk	8 ounces	300
Navy beans	1 cup	128
Okra	1/2 cup	50
Spinach, cooked	1/2 cup	122
Sweet potato, baked	1 medium	32
Swiss chard, cooked	1/2 cup	51
Tofu	1/2 cup	130
Turnip greens, cooked	1/2 cup	99
Yogurt	8 ounces	415

None of the above will help much if casein sensitivity is the issue. You're probably better off just swearing off the dairy, especially cheese. Every type of cheese has casein in it.

If you do drink milk or eat any dairy products, including cheese, yogurt, and butter, make sure it's organic. Factory-style large-scale dairy farms give cows growth hormones and antibiotics. Hormone additives seeping into dairy products have been linked to early puberty and sexual development in children who consume them. Antibiotic resistance in patients suffering from bacterial infections is a side effect linked to consuming products from cows treated with broad-spectrum antibiotics.

The calcium connection

You're probably wondering how you're supposed to get your calcium if you don't eat dairy products. Don't you need plenty of milk now to avoid thinning bones later in life? And what about your kids? Don't they need lots of milk for their growing bodies?

I get asked these questions all the time. The idea that drinking cow's milk is the best way to get the calcium you need for strong bones and for growing kids is myth. All around the world, most people can't digest milk and don't eat a lot of dairy products, yet the kids are healthy and the women have good bone health. In fact, a lot of scientific studies show an *inverse* relation between calcium and osteoporosis: Women in the countries that consume the most dairy have the *highest* osteoporosis rates. Despite how much milk we drink, American women over age 50 have one of the highest levels of hip fractures (an indicator of osteoporosis) in the world. The rate is exceeded only by Australia and New Zealand, where dairy consumption is even higher than in the United States.

It's possible that a diet high in protein from dairy foods offsets the calcium in them by causing an acid imbalance in the body. To neutralize the acidity, your body uses the calcium that normally circulates in your bloodstream; if that runs low, it pulls some from your bones. When you need a lot of calcium to counter acidity, you have less left for keeping your bones strong.

Bone strength comes from much more than just calcium, however. You also need to keep physically active, get enough vitamin D, and avoid alcohol and tobacco.

> Despite how much milk we drink, American women over age 50 have one of the highest levels of hip fractures, an indicator of osteoporosis, in the world.

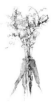

But back to dietary calcium. Lots of plant foods are rich in calcium, including beans and all those green leafy vegetables, like kale, spinach, and broccoli. Nuts, especially almonds, are another good source.

People who need to avoid dairy often ask me about taking calcium supplements. It's always better to get your nutrition from food, not pills, and some recent studies have linked calcium supplements to a sharply increased risk of heart disease in women. Better to fortify your bones with absorbable calcium from plant sources, so load up on kale and other dark, leafy greens every day. If you feel you still need a supplement, look for one made from plant sources such as kale and algae.

Soy

Although this Bad Boy is one of the most highly recommended foods for women, soy is another common offender when it comes to food intolerance—and despite the recommendations, it might not be good for women.

If you're soy intolerant, you don't produce the enzymes your body needs to break down the proteins in soy. That leads to symptoms such as cramping, abdominal pain, bloating, nausea, and diarrhea. A sure sign of soy intolerance is heartburn after eating soy foods. A lot of people are allergic to soy, although it usually takes a large amount to trigger a reaction. If you're allergic to soy and drink a big glass of soy milk, for instance, you might get hives, an itchy skin rash, or abdominal pain along with nausea, vomiting, or diarrhea. A small amount of soy sauce, however, probably wouldn't kick off a reaction.

Soy is often touted as a healthy plant protein that's a good substitute for meat or dairy foods. Today, soy is one of the largest agricultural crops in the United States. Unfortunately, most of the soy grown here is also genetically modified and highly subsidized. So, we now have a lot of cheap, genetically modified soy in our food supply. Soy is used in thousands of processed foods, often in hidden ways you'd never suspect. Unless you read the label very carefully, for example, you'd never know that soy is an important ingredient in a lot of energy bars, breakfast bars, and "nutrition" bars.

Soy is also the darling of many people who are eating a vegan or vegetarian diet or who want to avoid the cholesterol and saturated fat in meat. They buy soy products in place of animal protein. But are tofu (bean curd) hot dogs, sausages, burgers, and cheese really any better for you than their animal counterparts? Maybe not. Even if these products are made with 100 percent organic soybeans, the ingredients label sometimes shows that they're heavily processed and loaded with additives. Read your labels and buy products that contain only organic ingredients that you recognize.

There's a bigger problem than just the chemicals and taste of processed soy foods.

Soy contains phytoestrogens, meaning plant-based substances very similar to estrogen, the female hormone. So, if you eat a lot of soy foods, you're also getting a lot of phytoestrogens—and that may not be good for you. If you're a breast cancer patient whose tumor was estrogen sensitive, the last thing you would want to do is add something that mimics estrogen to your diet. If you're in perimenopause or menopause, soy phytoestrogens in the form of soy isoflavones are sometimes recommended as a natural treatment for hot flashes and other symptoms caused by your body's own diminishing supply of estrogen. These substances have the same problem as hormone-replacement therapy, however: a potential increase in your risk of breast cancer. Also, dietary soy has been linked to thyroid problems.

Needless to say, as a health coach I don't like to recommend something that could harm my clients. I suggest that all my female patients of any age eat soy foods only in moderation. If they have a history of thyroid problems, estrogen-sensitive breast cancer, or any other female cancer, I suggest actively avoiding soy foods. The exception would be small amounts of naturally fermented soy sauce or miso used for cooking.

But what about those reports from Asian countries that women who eat a lot of soy have *lower* rates of breast cancer and osteoporosis? Asian women eat soy mostly as soy sauce and fermented soy products, such as tempeh, miso, and natto. They do eat tofu in moderation, but they don't eat soy practically every day in the form of an additive to processed foods. They don't drink soy milk, much less eat soy cheese, soy ice cream, and soy burgers. When we look more closely at the claims that Asian women have less breast cancer and osteoporosis because of soy in the diet, they don't really hold up.

The bottom line on this Bad Boy is that he's powerful and carries a hormonal punch. If he's on your love list, make sure the soy you eat is organic, and enjoy it in its whole form, such as edamame (immature soy beans still in the pod) or organic tofu, only now and

> I suggest that all my female patients of any age eat soy foods only in moderation.

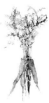

then. Use organic soy sauce and avoid excess processed soy, including soy milk (try almond or hemp milk instead). If you're avoiding soy on a doctor's recommendation, you must read every label on every item you add to your shopping cart, because soy is commonly found in many packaged foods—even in chocolate bars, candy, breakfast cereals, soups, and condiments.

Sugar

Look out, girl: This Bad Boy is highly addictive and will make you his love slave. This deadly Bad Boy has created an epidemic of obesity in unheard of proportions. It's in everything—80 percent of all processed foods have added sugar. Our palates have been so manipulated to crave sweetness that we Americans need it all day long.

Sugar is being force-fed to our children, disguised in cereal boxes and "healthy" drinks and energy bars. Because it's so addictive, if you need it, *you need it bad,* and that makes this Bad Boy really difficult to give up.

Sugar also messes with moods and energy. When we don't get it when we want it, we get depressed or irritable. Feed the sugar craving,

RICHARD   The Sugar Addict

Richard was married to one of my clients. After seeing how coaching helped her improve her diet, he scheduled a session with me as well. He told me he just wanted to tweak his already healthy diet. Richard was an athlete who worked out regularly and cared about his health. Although he was in great shape, he had been dealing with chronic joint pain since his late thirties. He felt the joint pain was genetic and that he couldn't do much about it.

It turned out that Richard's diet wasn't as healthy as he thought—and his chronic joint pain was optional.

Tutored by his wife, Richard drank protein smoothies daily and ate a well-balanced Flexible Vegetarian diet. His wife shopped for organic foods and cooked healthy meals each night.

When we went deeper into his health history, however, Richard casually mentioned candy. Almost

every day on his way home from work, he would feel so depleted that he would dash into a convenience store and grab a candy bar for a quick energy boost. We discussed better options for getting over that late-afternoon energy sag, like eating a piece of fruit along with a handful of nuts or having some hummus on whole-wheat crackers. Once he discovered some healthy snacks he liked, Richard was able to break his candy bar habit.

Breaking the habit had an unexpected side effect. Within a week, Richard had less pain in his joints. Within two weeks, his joint pain was gone. He called it a miracle, I called it reducing inflammation. When you sock your body with a big dose of refined sugar, it causes inflammation—and pain and swelling are classic symptoms. By removing the sugar, Richard had removed the source of his painful joint inflammation.

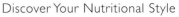

though, and hop on the energy rollercoaster—first the burst of energy, then the energy crash. For my clients, sugar means a midday energy slump, or a very strong need for something sweet after dinner, or cravings for candy, cookies, sweet snacks, soda, or a late afternoon glass of wine.

Unwanted weight gain is the most obvious side effect of sugar. Because of its addictive nature, it's nearly impossible to pass by the bowl of candy on your co-workers desk, or the leftover cookies in your fridge, or the cupcake store on the drive home, without at least thinking about having a taste. It can be really hard, as the urge is psychological as well as physical. Your body is signaling something you'd rather not hear, and sometimes it's screaming so loudly you cave in just to silence the cravings.

Fortunately, there are ways to satisfy your cravings for sweetness without adding sugar or pounds. You can still find pleasure in your food—this book isn't about deprivation, starvation, or never eating another cupcake.

MARIANNA   Sugar Is Sugar

Marianna was a self-described healthy eater, but she was also holding on to extra weight and not feeling as energized and bright as she needed to. She was a successful business owner with a lot of people dependent on her, and she found it frustrating that she didn't have this piece of her life figured out.

When she came to me for a nutritional consultation, we went through her usual diet. Like many of the people who contact me, she ate a lot of healthy food and made pretty good choices. I picked up on something right away, however, that told me why Marianna wasn't feeling fully energized.

Her daily diet was loaded with sugar, but not from white sugar and junk food. Marianna's diet was filled with fruit sugar, otherwise known as fructose. Every meal included or was followed by a sweet fruit. Her favorites were tropical fruits, especially bananas, pineapples, and mangos. During the day and in the evening she snacked on dried fruit.

Marianna thought that fruit was healthy and good for her. She had no idea that too much fruit could be the cause of her excess weight and sluggish energy levels.

I explained to Marianna that while fruit contains healthy fiber, phytochemicals, and phytonutrients, fructose is still a sugar. It was too much of the "good" sugar from the fruit that was affecting her energy level and causing her to bloat up and retain weight.

Marianna was shocked when I told her my theory, but she was game for a change. I gave her some enjoyable snack choices that weren't sugary, such as whole-grain organic crackers (Mary's Gone Crackers brand), low-sugar energy bars, and celery sticks spread with almond butter.

She immediately made the changes, tweaking her entire menu to remove most of the fruit. Her body's response supported my theory. She began to drop weight, almost effortlessly. It was clear that excess sugar from too much fruit had been the culprit.

Not all sweeteners send your blood sugar soaring and lead to a crash. You can have your cake and eat it, too, once you discover the right sweeteners.

Coconut sugar, also known as palm sugar, has a relatively low glycemic index (GI) ranking. The GI is a way of ranking foods by how quickly they make your blood sugar levels rise after eating them. Regular white table sugar has a GI rank of 100; coconut sugar is ranked at 35, meaning that it won't send your blood sugar rocketing up as soon as you eat it. Coconut sugar still has about the same number of calories as white sugar (16 per teaspoon).

Other natural sweeteners are also good choices, in moderation. White sugar has calories but no nutrition; natural sweeteners, especially if they're not heavily processed, bring some nutrition as well. Pure maple syrup, for instance, contains minerals such as manganese and zinc. Pure honey can help alleviate seasonal allergies in some people. Yacon syrup, made from the Andean tuber of the same name, gets its sweetness from fructooligosacchrides, which your body doesn't digest. That means you get a sweet flavor but fewer calories and less of a blood sugar spike. Stevia is a natural, intensely sweet sugar made from the leaves of a plant found in South America. A tiny bit goes a long way, so stevia has very little impact on your blood sugar. It's available as a powder or liquid; it's also sold in handy packets.

What about artificial sweeteners such as aspartame (NutraSweet, Equal), saccharine (Sweet 'N Low), and sucralose (Splenda)? They're even worse for you than sugar—think of them as the Bad Boy's evil Serial Killer twin. They're so bad for you that I'll discuss them separately later on in this chapter.

Caffeine

Caffeine is a drug that stimulates your central nervous system. You might not think that a cup of coffee is actually a drug delivery system, but it is. Does that make caffeine, something that's consumed daily by about 90 percent of the world's population, a Bad Boy? For some, yes; for others, no.

The most common sources of caffeine are coffee and tea; it's also found in chocolate, some herbal drinks, such as maté, and in cola drinks. It's even added to Mountain Dew soda, a good example of how a drug can legally be added to a food. And of course, caffeine is the energy in energy drinks.

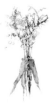

Caffeine can turn into a real Bad Boy when you get addicted to it. This isn't an addiction like heroin or even nicotine, but you can definitely become dependent on the caffeine boost. If you get a nasty headache, become irritable, or have trouble concentrating when you don't get your afternoon dose of coffee, for instance, you're dependent on it.

Being dependent on anything can affect your life in a negative way. People drink their coffee, energy drinks, or sodas for an energy and mood boost, but the effects are short-lived and last only four hours or so. After that, you're left wanting and needing that good mood back—you'll most likely reach for another energy hit. That can be a problem if the hit is coming from a sugary soda, energy drink, or coffee drink. You're adding a sugar high and crash to the caffeine effect.

Drinking caffeine boosts the brain's dopamine levels. Dopamine is the "feel good" neurotransmitter in your brain. That's why your morning coffee elevates your mood and prepares you to tackle the day in a wonderful way, and then throws you down a few hours later. You're wanting, needing, and craving more, and this Bad Boy then becomes so very addictive.

The real problem happens when coffee addiction leads to irritability and anxiety from being over-caffeinated. Think of the screaming mother with her coffee cup at the soccer game, or your snippy boss who threw that folder on the boardroom table. You most likely think your short moods or temper flare-ups are because of all the stress you're under, but caffeine might be gnawing away on your nervous system. If you get frequent headaches, muscle tension, gastrointestinal issues, or if you're easily dehydrated, you may want to check your caffeine consumption.

Caffeine addiction can make it difficult to fall asleep or stay asleep. Sleep is a non-negotiable necessity for your health and beauty, and if you're not getting seven or more hours a night, you're missing out. Cut out the caffeine for six hours before bedtime and you're likely to see a huge improvement in the quality and quantity of your sleep.

Caffeine isn't everybody's Bad Boy, especially if you keep your coffee consumption under control. In fact, caffeine has some definite health benefits. In the form of coffee, caffeine can promote gastrointestinal regularity, boost your brainpower and alertness, and help you function at peak intellectual levels. If you have a tension

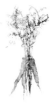

headache, the caffeine in a cup of coffee can help relieve the pain. There's even some evidence that coffee can cut your risk of liver and colorectal cancer.

Coffee is rich in antioxidants and minerals, and it's long been proven that the benefits of drinking tea outweigh the caffeine risks. This is where you need to be honest with yourself. We know you feel great when you have that morning coffee, but if you relate to any of the negative side effects mentioned here, it might be time to admit that caffeine is not going to be such a big part of your daily Nutritional Style. If you think you're drinking too much coffee (and have the acid stomach to prove it), try switching to gentler energy lifts, such as green, black, or white tea, yerba maté, or guayusa.

As for energy drinks and caffeine-laden sodas? They are true Serial Killers. Toss them from your kitchen. Ban them from your kids, and run, don't walk, when you see them coming.

The Serial Killers

These are the non-negotiable, cut-them-out-completely offenders to your health.

GMOs

Ted Bundy, one of the worst serial killers in history, looked normal. In fact, on the surface, he looked like a catch. College-educated, handsome, a gubernatorial appointee to a crime prevention unit in Seattle, enrolled in law school—what's not to like? Disarming and clever, he would lure women by asking for their help, sometimes wearing a cast to appear more helpless.

Genetically modified organisms (GMOs) are the Ted Bundy of the Serial Killer food lineup. Crops that are genetically modified and designed to resist pests and withstand the application of pesticides look and act normal. They blend in, but they pose a huge potential threat. All the money that goes into producing and marketing these foods doesn't change the fact we have no idea what permanent impacts we might face when we alter the genetic code of some of the world's largest and most essential crops. Today, most of the corn and soybeans grown in the United States come from genetically modified seeds. These GMOs then enter the food system as animal feed

> Coffee is rich in antioxidants and minerals, and it's long been proven that the benefits of drinking tea outweigh the caffeine risks.

or processed foods. Canola oil, widely used in processed foods, is almost always made with GMOs.

Worldwide, many nations have banned, regulated, or enforced labeling on GMOs. The most notable exceptions are the United States and Canada, which produce huge amounts of GMO crops unregulated by any government agency. Some states and municipalities have enacted laws requiring GMO labeling, but almost all consumers are on their own.

GMOs carry a number of environmental and health risks. The American Academy of Environmental Medicine (AAEM) has tested GMO foods and reported that "several animal studies indicate serious health risks associated with Genetically Modified (GM) food, including infertility, immune system problems, accelerated aging, faulty insulin regulation, and changes in major organs and the gastrointestinal system." They asked physicians to advise patients to avoid GM foods. FDA scientists have warned that GM foods could create hard-to-detect side effects, such as allergies, new diseases, and nutritional issues.

GMOs have been around since the 1980s, which is long enough for a lot of good research to show how dangerous they are. Numerous studies in scientific journals continue to document the health problems these crops can cause. Among other issues, GM crops have been modified to withstand the powerful herbicide Roundup, produced by Monsanto. That means GM crops contain Roundup— but eating this stuff has been shown to cause infertility, mammary tumors, kidney damage, and liver damage in animals. The effects of GMOs on humans are likely to be just as serious as they are on rats, but they'll take a lot longer to become obvious.

GMOs are potentially the worst of the worst of the non-negotiable foods for your diet. The unknowns and untested risks involved place them at the top of my list. In just ten to fifteen years, GMOs have infiltrated our food supply. In the average U.S. supermarket, thousands of the food items contain GM ingredients. One big reason the United States doesn't demand that food producers label GM foods is that the majority of products lining the inner aisles of the grocery stores—the packages, mixes, soups, cereals, prepared meals, breads, condiments, snacks, pastas, and more—contain GM ingredients. Big agriculture fears that bringing this to light with forced labeling has the potential to damage sales and hurt the economy.

> Worldwide, many nations have banned, regulated, or enforced labeling on GMOs. The most notable exceptions are the United States and Canada.

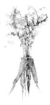

The European Union led the way with laws demanding labeling in 1998, followed by Japan, New Zealand and Australia, China, South Korea, Saudi Arabia, Thailand, Indonesia, Russia, India, Chile, Taiwan, and South Africa. As of 2014, the United States and Canada, two giant producers of GM crops, remained conspicuously absent from this list. Many states in the United States are taking action and have initiated bills that will require GMO labeling.

The biggest environmental concern with GM crops is cross-contamination. Non-GM fields are being cross-pollinated by neighboring GM fields. Traditional farmers who don't want to use GM seeds they must buy from a few massive corporations only are forced to watch as their once untainted crops develop into fields of genetically modified plants. GMOs are the genie let out of the bottle—untested, unreliable, and spreading with no means of containment.

Pesticides

You could say that pesticide use has made vegetables and fruits even better than before. Pesticides keep off the insects, fungi, and other pests that mar the ideal shape and color of these foods. Without a spot to mar their perfect skin, in season and out, pesticide-treated produce is beautiful, but dangerously so.

Think of the red, round tomato you find at the grocery store in the middle of winter, or the perfectly red, perfectly shaped apples you see year-round. Flawless beauty is deceiving. Heavy doses of various insecticides, fungicides, and other chemicals give these foods their perfect outward appearance. In addition to their very serious impact on the environment, all these assorted pesticides get into you when you eat foods that have been treated with them. This is true even if you wash them—residues remain. The toxins in pesticides are linked to a variety of health issues, including brain and nervous system toxicity, cancer, hormone disruption, and skin, eye, and lung irritation. Depending on the fruit or vegetable, more than 100 different chemicals can be left as residue when you eat it, even after washing. Think about that the next time you grab a bag of conventionally grown celery.

The best way to avoid pesticides is to choose organic produce whenever possible. They may not look as nice, but I prefer my oddly shaped heirloom tomato varieties in season to the plump, plastic, tasteless kind in the winter. I'm not bothered by the looks of surprise I get when I bring my organic heirloom corn to the table, complete

The lists below were compiled by the Environmental Working Group as a guide to choosing the worst and best foods in terms of pesticide residues. The worst foods should be avoided if organic varieties aren't available; the best foods are acceptable if organic varieties aren't available.

The Dirty Dozen Plus

1. apples
2. celery
3. cherry tomatoes
4. cucumber
5. grapes
6. hot peppers
7. nectarines (imported)
8. peaches
9. potatoes
10. spinach
11. strawberries
12. sweet bell peppers

Plus: collards, kale, summer squash, and zucchini

The Clean Fifteen

1. asparagus
2. avocado
3. cabbage
4. cantaloupe
5. corn
6. eggplant
7. grapefruit
8. kiwi
9. mangoes
10. mushrooms
11. onions
12. papayas
13. pineapples
14. sweet peas (frozen)
15. sweet potatoes

with pieces cut out where the worms got in. I'll take the holey, misshapen bushel of apples off the tree in my backyard over those perfectly formed shiny red ones that taste like soap.

Organic produce is more expensive, however, and it's not always easy to find. The wonderful folks at the nonprofit organization Environmental Working Group produce annual lists of the Dirty Dozen Plus and the Clean 15. The Dirty Dozen identifies the produce you must avoid if it's not organic. These fruits and vegetables are heavily sprayed and when tested contained the highest levels of pesticide residue. The Clean 15 lists produce that is safe to eat even if it's not organic.

I often hear that buying organic food is too expensive; shopping with the Clean 15 in mind is a great way to save money. But don't skimp on your health—avoid the Dirty Dozen at all costs. There's a wonderful saying that goes, "Pay the farmer, or pay the doctor." At some point, you will pay with health problems for eating high concentrations of pesticide residues.

Organic growing methods support and enrich the soil. Organic farmers often use crop rotation and plant a variety of crops to ensure that the soil stays fertile naturally, without chemical fertilizers, and isn't depleted of its vital minerals. Eating organically supports not only your health, but our earth as well.

Many people believe that organic food tastes better, and those used to eating only organic foods can taste the difference. Food writer and scientist Harold McGee explains why. He says that because organic produce isn't protected by pesticides, the plants are constantly under attack from bugs and blights of all kinds. This sounds like a bad thing, but it's not.

When plants are under attack, they begin to ramp up production of their chemical defenses. For us, these "defenses" translate directly into flavor and aroma. McGee says, "Because they're not protected by pesticides, organic plants that suffer from insect attack can accumulate higher levels of flavor chemicals and other protective molecules, including antioxidants." Plants under attack by pests become heartier. Heartier plants mean more flavor and nutrition.

Think about the last time you picked a luscious autumn apple right off a tree or plucked a fresh spring strawberry from the ground. Compare that memory to the bland, mealy apples you often buy at the grocery store, or the tasteless strawberries they sell. Nothing is like

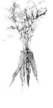

fresh organic food that's in season, and in this book I want you to discover the pleasures of eating this way.

Mystery foods

Many people say, "I don't eat processed foods," yet their cupboards are stocked with breakfast cereals (yes, even organic, gluten-free and fat-free ones are processed, often with added sugar), energy bars, cans of soup, tomato sauce, pastas, crackers, and chips. Frozen pizza and ice cream fill their freezers.

Processed foods aren't just convenience foods. While some processed foods are better than others, you'll want to be discerning when it comes to the processed foods lining the inner aisles of the grocery store. Serial Killers lurk there in the brightly colored boxes and cans and packages that scream, "Choose me!"

Food processing is now a large part of our food economy, with artificial sweeteners giving us an unnatural craving for sweets all day long, and food-coloring chemicals that are linked to everything from cancer to allergies, including hyperactivity, autism, and tumors, according to researchers at the Center for Science in the Public Interest (CSPI).

Common preservatives are linked to liver and kidney damage, growth retardation, and cancer. The worst part is that food manufacturers are mainly self-regulating. As consumers, we're left to trust the food conglomerates of America to decide our food safety without oversight. Foods bearing the phrase "natural flavors," for example, can contain toxins that can harm your health, yet most people see that deceiving phrase and believe the product is good for them.

Your grocery store can seem like a minefield, and it's hard to know whom, and what, to trust. As a general rule, avoid foods that contain numerous ingredients that are unrecognizable or impossible to pronounce. If you don't know what calcium propionate is or why it's on the ingredients label, it's a good idea to skip that product.

Some processed foods are definitely better than others. In fact, I use some organic processed foods in my own kitchen because they're convenient, free of additives, and taste great. Processed foods labeled as certified organic are a much better choice. The organic label means they don't contain unsafe additives. For example, cheese crackers are a processed food and a bestseller with moms everywhere as a tasty snack for kids. The organic version is a much healthier choice than the nonorganic because it doesn't have as many preservatives and other additives. The organic version is still a processed food and still not the best snack choice for kids, but at least it's not a Serial Killer. A piece of dried (sulfite-free) fruit, or a handful of nuts or pumpkin seeds would be a much healthier choice, but hey, life isn't perfect. Sometimes your kids just want to crunch on a cheesy snack, like all the other kids. I'm a mom and I definitely get that. Although organic processed foods are healthier than the conventional brands, by far, it's not an invitation to load up on them. Use them wisely, to add fun to a lunchbox or as an occasional treat.

The same principle applies to gluten-free processed foods. They aren't necessarily healthy, they just don't contain gluten. Likewise, low-fat and fat-free processed foods aren't necessarily healthy either; they just have less fat. They don't even always have fewer calories: reduced-fat Oreos have the same calorie count as regular Oreos!

When food manufacturers take fat out of their products, they replace it with sugar, the baddest of the Bad Boys. Because these foods lack the fat that makes you feel satisfied, they are not only made sweeter, they also don't fill you up as much and you end up eating more. Now you have a sugar habit, still crave fat, and need to detox from the added chemicals you've just taken in.

You need healthy fat from your food to survive and thrive (I'll talk about this a lot more in chapter nine). In my experience as a nutrition coach, the increase of fat-free food offerings in the supermarket over the last couple of decades has led to an entire generation of women who have digestive issues, constipation being number one on the list.

Factory-farmed animal protein

Just as non-organic produce is heavily sprayed and toxic, factory-farmed meats and poultry are raised on non-organic feed laced with hormones and antibiotics. If you eat a lot of this stuff, you may eventually develop antibiotic resistance and get overloaded with excess hormones. Factory farming has created a Serial Killer food that strikes in the most insidious of ways, masquerading as a necessary protein to unsuspecting people everywhere.

Children in the United States and the developed world are reaching puberty much earlier than in previous generations. Young girls often now develop signs of puberty—budding breasts and body hair—at age eight or younger and begin menstruation before age ten.

> When food manufacturers take fat out of their products, they replace it with sugar, the baddest of the Bad Boys.

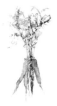

Many researchers feel the excess calories most kids now consume, combined with the hormones they're getting from meat, poultry, and milk, have a lot to do with earlier puberty. It's also possible that the many hormone-disrupting chemicals in the environment, such as the BPA found in some plastics, have something to do with it.

Most animal proteins in the United States come from factory farming, a nightmarish practice that began in the 1920s and has gradually worsened since. Chickens and hogs are bred in close, tightly confined indoor quarters without proper air and ventilation or sanitation. They are often sick and are routinely given antibiotics to ensure their "health."

As seen in the movie *Food, Inc.*, factory-farmed chickens are raised in a toxic, closed environment and fed hormones to fatten them faster. Factory-bred cows often stand in their own excrement, penned in close proximity to one another. They often can't move because they are packed in so closely, and they don't have access to grass or fields. The animals are frequently sick, and if you were to witness this scene you'd imagine them to be miserable. Their meat is sold at your grocery store, and you're consuming the energy of that mistreated animal.

As you learn more about what's in your food, and how everything you put in your mouth affects you, you'll want to become more discerning about what you take in. Remember, you are what you eat. If the cow led a terrible, tortured life, or even died a torturous death, that animal's stress hormones were high, and you're taking in all that negativity and pain when you eat it.

If you do choose to eat meat or animal proteins of any kind, including chicken, beef, or eggs, choose the humanely raised organic version—raised without hormones or high amounts of antibiotics. Choose the meat that roamed as it was meant to roam, or grazed as it was meant to graze, eating food that it was meant to eat. That's the meat you're meant to eat, not an adulterated, stressed-out version that's raised in a factory. (See sources for healthier animal proteins in the resources section of this book.)

Artificial sweeteners

Like most Serial Killers, artificial sweeteners can be charming and deceiving. They seem harmless enough, but these guys are dangerous—and pervasive. This is the one non-negotiable change I have with my clients. If you're hooked on diet soda, you're coming off it, now. I've helped wean many people off this dangerous drug, masked as a good guy, and they still thank me for it.

Artificial sweeteners are also known as noncaloric sugar substitutes. They're used instead of sucrose (table sugar) to sweeten foods and beverages without adding calories. The most commonly used artificial sweeteners are aspartame (NutraSweet, Equal), saccharine (Sweet 'N Low), sucralose (Splenda), acesulfame-K (Sunette), and neotame, an even sweeter version of aspartame.

You know them as the pink, yellow, and blue packets that are everywhere you go. They're in every restaurant, diner, break room, and maybe even on your own kitchen table. I was at a party where these pretty packets were displayed like a colorful fan. I'm sure the caterers were proud of their artistic presentation, but I wanted to mess it up and run away. I didn't—good manners, and the knowledge that more would surely appear to replace them, held me back.

The Center for Science in the Public Interest (CSPI) cautions consumers to avoid aspartame, saccharine, and acesulfame-K because they're unsafe in even the normal amounts consumed.

Aspartame is particularly concerning because it contains phenylalanine (50 percent), aspartic acid (40 percent), and methanol (10 percent), three well-recognized neurotoxins. These neurotoxins create excitotoxicity in your brain cells. Among other things, neurotoxins are linked to brain diseases such as Parkinson's and Alzheimer's.

Consuming aspartame regularly is linked to headaches, migraines, dizziness, insomnia, hyperactivity, anxiety, heart arrhythmias, and mood swings.

A number of very strong scientific studies show a link between artificial sweeteners and weight *gain,* the opposite of the desired effect! More than one recent study has shown that people who switched to diet soda from regular soda gained weight. Is that gorgeous actress with the rockin' body featured on the label and in the advertising *really* drinking diet soda every day? I'll venture to say that she keeps her gorgeous body by drinking it only at the photo shoot.

Artificial sweeteners are also linked to sugar cravings—your body never quite gets what it believes it's going to get with artificial sweeteners. They leave your body wanting the real thing. The next thing you know, you're face-planted in a carton of ice cream at 10:00 p.m. It's all over.

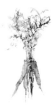

I worked with a young guy named Bradley who had spent years addicted to diet soda. He was almost one hundred pounds overweight and had tried every diet known to man. I had him read an article on the dangerous side effects of artificial sweeteners. It made a profound difference in his life. Realizing that he was pouring a chemical into his body and causing his own cells to act crazy was enough to scare Bradley out of his addiction.

Bradley dropped the toxic sugar-free drinks and began to lose a lot of weight almost without trying. He lost his out-of-control cravings for sugar—cravings he had believed he was quenching with diet soda. The reality was that his cravings were still there; he was binge eating on sugary foods every evening. Despite his diet soda habit, Bradley steadily gained weight all through his twenties.

Giving up diet soda wasn't easy for Bradley, but I weaned him off the addictive brown drink slowly, substituting lots of healthy drinks that he loved. The end result was that with the toxic sugar

MEGAN | Artificial Sweeteners: The Devil in Action

Megan was having trouble losing weight even though she was sticking closely to her weight-loss diet. She had chosen a good plan with lots of variety and was now eating plenty of healthy salads and clean foods. Megan enjoyed cooking, so she was preparing her meals herself.

Megan contacted me in frustration. Despite her positive dietary changes, she had reached a plateau. She couldn't figure out why she was holding on to those last ten pounds.

We carefully went through her menus and her daily routine. Megan worked out several times a week and her meals were excellent. I began to think that perhaps she wasn't telling me everything. After more investigation on my part, she casually mentioned that she hated drinking water; instead, she drank "a few" cans of diet soda every day. I asked, "How many, exactly?" She responded, "Oh, four or five, maybe six."

Megan was addicted to the sweet taste of diet soda and to the lift she got from the caffeine. She didn't realize that artificial sweeteners are among the most dangerous of liaisons. When I shared the details with her and pointed out how toxic diet sodas are, she really didn't want to hear it. With great reluctance, she agreed to cut back on her diet sodas. For the first few days, she cut back to just three cans. To replace the diet sodas, she drank plain water with a splash of lemon and a pinch of stevia. It wasn't easy, but within a few weeks Megan had weaned herself off the diet sodas completely.

At that point, she felt better overall, had more energy, and was significantly less bloated. She dropped a few pounds right away just from losing the bloat. As she added more water to support her metabolism, those last ten pounds finally budged—they were gone within a few more weeks. By giving up the diet sodas, Megan also found that her skin was clearer and had a nice glow. Although she still sometimes misses her diet sodas, Megan tells me she'll never go back to them.

substitutes out his system, he finally felt like a young person. He was able to get back into the dating scene, soda free.

The FDA doesn't recognize the link between these sweet Serial Killers and anything harmful, so it's up to you to stand up for yourself here. Drop the pink, blue, and yellow packets now and find an organic stevia packet instead. You may have to carry those around, but who cares? That and your taser will protect you from any Serial Killer you might come across. Tell this artificially sweet guy, "Back off, Buster, or I'll be comin' at you with seven kinds of smoke!"

Trans fats

Trans fats are like a Serial Killer at large. He's wanted in several states, yet until very recently he roamed free and undetected in our nation's food supply. Fortunately, in 2013 he was finally apprehended by the FDA and banned.

For decades before that, trans fats (also called partially hydrogenated vegetable oils) were a common ingredient in fast foods, snack foods and baked goods, and a lot of processed foods.

Trans fats are made by processing cheap vegetable oil with hydrogen. The end result is a type of fat that has a longer shelf life and holds up better to heat than regular vegetable oil.

The problem with trans fats is that the fat molecules are altered beyond recognition by your body. When you eat trans fats, your digestive system says, "Huh? What is this stuff? What enzymes am I supposed to use to digest this?" And because you can't make digestive enzymes that break trans fats down completely, they end up circulating in your bloodstream in the form of tiny, artery-clogging fat drops called triglycerides.

For years, doctors and scientists pointed out the risks of trans fats: heart disease, stroke, diabetes, obesity, and more. Eventually, the FDA changed the rules so that manufacturers had to list trans fats on the food information label. There was a loophole big enough to drive a heart-lung machine through, though: If a serving had 0.5 grams or less of trans fats, the label could call it zero instead. Consumers were unknowingly still getting hefty doses of trans fats from doughnuts, cookies, pizza, and other processed foods. They were also getting plenty of trans fats from the oil in the deep fryers used for french fries, fried fish, and other fast foods. Gradually, due to

> So now you're wondering, how do I begin to figure this stuff out? How do I learn what my Nutritional Style is? I invite you to get started by trying a cleanse.

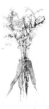

regulation and public awareness, these Serial Killers started to show up less in food, especially processed foods in your grocery store.

Now that trans fats have finally been banned, you have one less Serial Killer to worry about.

So now you're wondering, how do I begin to figure this stuff out? How do I learn what my Nutritional Style is? I invite you to get started by trying a cleanse. Not a rigid, starvation diet kind of cleanse, but several meals a day of delicious, nutrient-rich foods that will fortify and strengthen you. Cleansing will help to clear your body of toxins so that clarity of thought, and knowing what works for you, can come through. You'll love being able to hear what your body has been trying to tell you for years.

Join me for the Nutritional Style Cleanse.

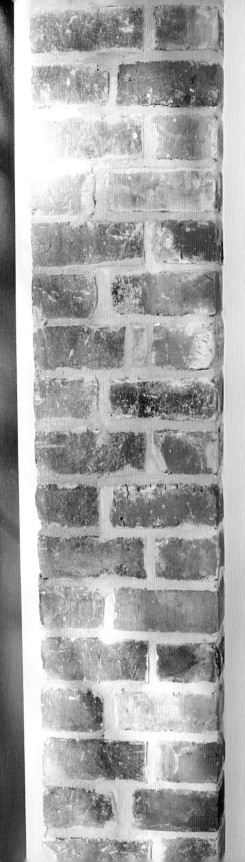
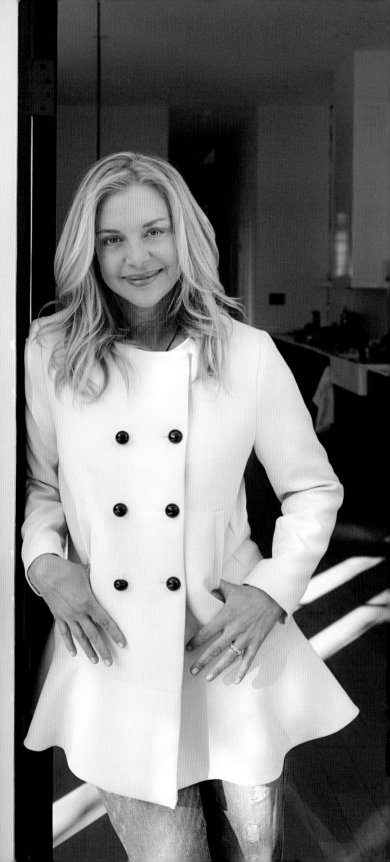

CHAPTER FOUR

Cleansing in Style

Finding your cleansing style, just like finding your Nutritional Style, is a wonderful way to help maintain optimal health and keep your body finely tuned, on point, and brimming with energy.

Why should you think about spending some time on a whole-foods detoxifying diet twice a year? Because living in today's modern world makes cleansing essential. We take in toxins from our environment through the air we breathe, whatever touches our skin, and the food we eat. Our bodies' normal detoxifying organs, especially the liver, colon, kidneys, and skin (did you know your skin is your body's largest organ?) can become overwhelmed by all they have to do. Sometimes they need a break, which is where detoxing comes in.

Even if you eat 100 percent organic food all the time, you'll still benefit from cleansing—toxins come at us from all directions, not just our food. And a cleanse is a fantastic way to kick off a new lifestyle and way of eating, or to take a break from indulgences that you may have enjoyed a little too often.

A cleanse is a good way to spring clean your body after the less active winter months, when the weather keeps you indoors and a little too close to the refrigerator. I suggest doing a cleanse early in the spring, when the weather begins to warm and the days are getting longer. A second cleanse in the late fall, as the days cool off and get shorter, gets you ready for the long winter ahead.

A cleanse is not a diet.
A cleanse is the beginning of a new way of thinking and living in this world.

A Cleanse Is Not a Diet

While weight loss can be one nice side effect of cleansing, it's not the goal. A cleanse is not a diet. A cleanse is the beginning of a new way of thinking and living in this world. Most diets are restrictive and prohibitive, a setup for failure. When you come off your diet, you still don't know how to eat nutritiously to sustain your weight loss. Diets also can leave you feeling lousy, because most of them don't promote eating life-enhancing foods. If you go on a diet that insists you buy its diet-food meals or food packets to mix with water, or take its powders or pills and follow a rigid set of instructions, you won't be eating in a well-balanced, healthy way, much less eating according to your personal Nutritional Style. Most diets—such as those that eliminate or severely restrict carbohydrates—omit vital elements of nutrition. By definition, a diet creates a feeling of missing out or denial. You cause yourself unnecessary anxiety worrying about whether you're doing the diet "right" or whether you'll get to enjoy good food again.

The cleanse I offer to my clients adds greater amounts of healthy, life-enhancing foods and removes toxic or potentially toxic foods from your daily consumption.

Toxic foods and substances cause inflammation. Let's digress a bit and explain what I mean. Imagine you're in your kitchen slicing up some veggies. The knife slips and you cut your finger. You swear, reach for a paper towel to stop the bleeding, wash off the cut, put on a bandage, maybe look around for some sympathy, and get back to work. Later on, you notice the area is a bit red, a bit swollen, feels a bit warm, and *hurts.* Those are the markers of inflammation—your immune system is releasing all sorts of natural chemicals to heal the damage and kill off any germs that might have entered the area. In a few days your finger heals up and the inflammation goes away.

But what if the source of the inflammation never really goes away? What if your diet is consistently high in inflammatory foods, such as sugar or gluten, or if you're constantly exposed to toxins, such as pesticides or air pollution? In that case, the inflammation can become chronic. You still have the redness, warmth, and swelling that characterize inflammation, but they're happening inside your body, where you can't see or feel them directly. Chronic inflammation works away silently, damaging your blood vessels, your organs,

> The cleanse I offer to my clients adds greater amounts of healthy, life-enhancing foods and removes toxic or potentially toxic foods from your daily consumption.

your skin, your brain—every part of your body. Inflammation is the root cause of most of the major chronic diseases in the United States today. It plays a role in cancer, heart disease, brain deterioration, diabetes, high blood pressure, asthma, sinus infection, and many other diseases of modern society.

If you eat inflammatory foods on a regular basis, or are frequently exposed to toxins, such as fumes from the carpeting in your office, your body is continually reacting. If you keep on alert like this, day after day, your immune system may begin to attack healthy cells. This might show up as a rash or achy joints, or possibly as an autoimmune disease such as rheumatoid arthritis, or in the worst case, as cancer, when cells grow rapidly and out of control. Even if you don't have any visible signs of an immune system running in the red zone, chronic inflammation can make you feel exhausted, foggy, or depressed.

Removing inflammatory foods during the cleanse allows your body to cool down and rest, so your cells can eliminate toxins that have built up over time. This also gives your liver, kidneys, colon, and skin a bit of a break—they don't have to work so hard detoxifying your body.

More important, a cleanse is a way to get yourself off inflammatory foods for good. In my experience, people who do a cleanse feel so much better afterward that they don't want to go back to eating the sugary junk foods and other bad stuff. They'd rather stick with the whole foods, juices, and other energizing foods they ate during the cleanse and add in other healthy delights.

Our Toxic World

Genetically modified crops, foods heavily sprayed with pesticides and herbicides, meat full of antibiotics and hormones, and air and water pollution continuously assault our bodies. Most homes, schools, and offices are built with chemically treated lumber and materials, and decorated with carpets and furniture treated with toxic chemicals. Even the flimsy receipt from the supermarket is treated with a toxic chemical linked to cancer. Our lives are filled with electronic devices that contain toxic heavy metals and have screens that emit eye-damaging blue light Try as you can to avoid

The signs that your body would appreciate a cleanse are numerous, but they can vary considerably from person to person. If you're consistently having one or more of the signs listed here, think about doing a cleanse, even if it's just for a few days. Your body will thank you.

Skin and Hair

Dry skin
Itchy or scaly skin
Pimples or acne
Broken blood vessels
Dry hair
Thinning hair
Brittle nails

Headaches

Daily headaches
Migraines
Sinus headaches and infections

Digestion

Bloating
Constipation
Diarrhea

Body and Joints

Aching joints
Body aches
Inability to exercise for long
Low energy

Brain

Depression
Fuzzy thinking (brain fog)
Insomnia
Mood swings

them, unnatural chemicals are everywhere. A cleanse allows your body to release some of these accumulated toxins.

Benefits of Cleansing

Cleansing is a way to flush toxins from your body. Even though the body does this naturally, the cleansing organs—liver, kidneys, intestines, colon, and skin—are overworked under the constant strain of living in a toxic environment and eating processed foods. Cleansing gives the body a rest, and also can improve blood sugar imbalances. Other annoying problems, such as dry, itchy, or scaly skin, headaches or migraines, allergies, weight gain, sleeplessness, and even depression, often improve during and after a cleanse. Cleansing can give you gorgeous skin, and a healthy glow that will make your friends wonder what you've been doing.

Many of us suffer from what the medical establishment refers to as minor medical ailments—a runny nose, seasonal allergies, eczema, bloating, headache, or sinus congestion—that can be helped or eliminated by cleansing. Doctors often tell you to treat these issues with over-the-counter pills, sprays, or creams that mask the symptoms but never get to the root cause. Regardless of what new pharmaceuticals emerge, without treating the cause, you're facing a lifetime of dependence on over-the-counter medications that add to the toxicity in your body.

Do You Need to Cleanse?

Cleansing is a great way to clear up minor symptoms now that could lead to bigger, harder-to-fix symptoms later. After working with a lot of clients over the years, I've found that five common symptoms usually mean you need to clear out the toxins.

You're bloated

Eating foods that are high in bad fats, sugar, and gluten if you're sensitive, leads to indigestion and bloating. Over time, this affects your gut health. Your digestive tract is home to 70 percent of your overall immunity. If you're not doing well in this area, your overall health suffers. A cleanse helps to flush your gut of bad bacteria, lets your intestinal lining heal from any gluten damage, and gets things moving smoothly. End result? A less bloated appearance.

You're irritable, moody, and finding it difficult to cope with stress

Stress and moodiness can be a sign that you're toxic; your body is challenged by trying to eliminate too many toxins. In other words, it can't keep up.

Eating a standard American diet filled with processed foods, eating non-organic foods filled with antibiotics, hormones, and pesticides, or drinking too much alcohol or caffeine can lead to toxicity even if you indulge only now and then. Cleansing clears those toxins out, in a gentle way.

One of the biggest side effects of cleansing is a sense of CALM. Nice, huh?

Dull skin or break-outs

If your body is congested with toxicity, it can actually prevent nutrients from reaching your skin. Your skin is the window to your health, and dull, lifeless and off-color skin can be an indication that your diet is not ideal, or that there are toxins that need to be flushed out.

One of the biggest benefits of cleansing is clear, glowing skin. You often see that phrase associated with cleansing—because it's TRUE.

Cleanse for just two weeks and you'll be thinking, maybe for the first time in a long time, "I have gorgeous skin!"

Brain fog

An inability to focus is blamed on a lot of things these days: adult ADD, computer use overload, or aging. What's often forgotten is that toxicity in your body fogs your brain and slows your mental prowess down.

Cleansing clears out your brain fog and gives you clarity and a sharpness that you thought was gone forever. Get ready for that new career!

Puffy eyes

This one is the "tell" in my mirror. When I wake up with puffy eyes or bags under my eyes after a vacation, or a few weeks of too many parties, I know that I'm carrying toxins that need to be eliminated.

Puffy eyes can indicate overloaded liver or kidneys, two organs that are an integral part of the elimination process. Cleansing can give you back years of aging, just in the eyes alone!

Cleansing Basics

A cleanse is more than just following a set of dietary instructions for a few weeks. To be successful, a cleanse must involve education, learning, and self-discovery—or you'll go right back to your old habits. The cleanse plan I teach my clients is rooted in consuming whole foods, so you can learn how to feed yourself well and get good nutrition during the cleanse. My goal is to open your eyes to how certain foods and food groups may be affecting your overall health.

Cleansing according to my plan allows your body to adjust to new foods gradually, as you slowly add them in. After your cleanse you'll be able to discover which inflammatory foods are affecting you negatively as you add them back into your diet.

The Duration of the Cleanse

For most of my clients, I recommend a two-week cleanse, preceded by a week to ease in to it, and followed by a week to ease out. I call this the 1-2-1 schedule because you need to keep in mind that the weeks before and after cleansing are just as important as the two weeks spent on it. This 1-2-1 schedule will provide the healthiest, most gentle, and most effective cleanse, with results that last.

A two-week main cleanse is ideal for detoxification. Two weeks is about right for allowing your body rest and recovery time as it detoxifies. If you can't go this long, still allow time to ease off your cleanse—ideally take up to a week so that your body can adjust.

I ask my clients to remove the inflammatory foods listed in the chart on page 65 for the two weeks of the cleanse period. In the week before you begin the cleanse, gradually cut back on these foods. Most people take about three to five days to adjust to the cleanse, but if you prepare your body the week prior and begin to remove or cut down on some of these foods, you'll have an easier time once you begin. If you want to return any of these foods to your diet after the cleanse, ease them back in—and if possible, cut back permanently on them.

Cravings while Cleansing

Dairy, sugar, coffee, and processed foods, including breads and pasta, can be addictive. Your body wasn't designed to eat any of these foods as frequently as most people today do. Food manufacturers knowingly add ingredients like sugar in various forms to a lot of packaged and prepared foods to make them more flavorful—and addictive. Be prepared as you enter your cleanse. The cravings may kick in big time once you've removed some of your favorite foods.

Cravings should not be ignored or resisted. A cleanse is a great time to get in touch with your cravings and to realize how addicted you are. Some people will have a hard time not having a candy bar every day or a tall, foamy latte each morning. Your body reacts to

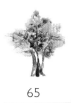

INFLAMMATORY FOODS TO AVOID

Sugar	Especially avoid refined white sugar. This includes the sugar additives used in processed foods, such as fructose, high fructose corn syrup, and any sugars other than those on the cleansing foods list found on pages 68 and 69.
Gluten	Found in most breads, crackers, snack foods, and many processed foods.
Dairy	Includes milk, cheese, butter, and even yogurt for the duration of the cleanse.
Alcohol	All spirits, beer, and wine. Your pancreas will thank you, as this will help to stabilize blood sugar levels. Most people experience lighter moods and more even energy levels throughout the day because of this change. Do this only if you'll enjoy looking ten years younger when you're done.
Processed foods	This means all the bags and boxes in your cupboard, including most pasta, breads, energy bars, snack packages, boxed cereals, crackers, or anything with multiple ingredients. Basically, if it's in a package, it has to go.
Soy foods	This includes tofu, edamame, tempeh, and imitation soy products such as soy milk and soy ice cream. Many think of soy as a health food, but it can be inflammatory for some people. Removing soy during the cleanse will help you find out if soy is a problem.
Coffee	Although coffee has some health benefits, if you are intolerant of it, the benefits do not outweigh the harm. To avoid caffeine withdrawal headaches, ease off the coffee slowly; drink black or green tea instead.

these foods in the same way it responds to opiate drugs, triggering the brain to release "feel good" endorphins or the hormone dopamine.

Don't think of the cleanse as starving or self-denial. Remember the dangerous liaisons and how those Bad Boys lure you in. Use your cravings to find out what you really want. For example, craving dairy could have an emotional component—the craving may indicate you need more affection and hugs. Or on the physical level, your body might need more calcium, so it's looking for dairy. On the cleanse, you'll discover better ways to get calcium your body can use through kale, chard, and other leafy green sources.

Switch your thinking to a sense of abundance and adding in. Add healthy substitutes *before* you lose out to your cravings, and learn what your body truly needs in the process.

If you follow the prep week tips listed below you'll be ready to handle those pesky cravings. Having healthy alternative foods on hand will help you quash cravings before they hit. (See the Easy Substitutions chart below.)

Greens, as a smoothie, a green juice, or a salad are a fantastic food to balance out your body's nutrition and diminish cravings. Adding in greens, in whatever way you like, will help to gradually erase the need for processed, salty, sweet, or creamy foods.

The Nutritional Style Cleanse: Prep Week

For prep week, begin to reduce your intake of foods from the inflammatory foods list. Do not eliminate them yet, but reduce the amount

EASY SUBSTITUTIONS

If you eat this . . .	try this instead
breakfast sandwich	oatmeal with nuts, almond milk, and cinnamon
Greek yogurt	smoothie, green ice cream (see the recipe on page 182)
bread	brown rice, quinoa, or millet pilaf
potato chips or pretzels	kale chips (see the recipe on page 191), roasted chickpeas, sweet potato fries (see the recipe on page 188)
candy bar	dark chocolate bar made with natural sweetener
coffee	green tea or low-caffeine tea, or coffee substitute
wine	sparkling water with lemon

you consume on a daily basis. If you eliminate these foods too fast, you'll begin cleansing under stress. Prep week is about *slowly* preparing your body. Jumping into a cleanse from a processed diet or a diet high in animal proteins can be painful, and unless you ease off in advance, you could feel sick, exhausted, and unhappy when you begin.

Even if you would define your diet as good, you'll be thankful if you take some time to allow your body to adjust to a cleaner diet.

Ideally, allow seven days for your preparation; if you can't do a whole week, do at least three and preferably five days. Use the easy substitutions chart on page 66 to help you start easing in to the cleanse phase.

PREP WEEK AT A GLANCE

As you get ready for the main part of your cleanse, follow these tips for easing in.

Remove heavy animal proteins in favor of lighter ones

Beef can have a long transit time in your digestion, creating more work for your body. Removing beef and pork several days before your cleanse is easy to do and will allow your digestion to begin to lighten up. Go for wild-caught fish or poultry instead.

Ease up on alcohol

Alcohol is high in carbohydrates and creates inflammation. It also feeds yeast in your gut and creates a puffy appearance. And, of course, it can be addictive. If you drink liquor, wine, or beer on a regular basis, stop as you prepare for the cleanse. You can dilute your drink with more water or dilute your wine as a spritzer; if you prefer beer, it's best to just eliminate it for now.

Cut back on caffeine

Quitting coffee cold turkey is tough, and could leave you grumpy, anxious, and with a bad headache. Go easy and wean off of the dark stuff the week before your cleanse. Try removing half a cup a day as you go.

Cut back on processed bread and crackers in favor of whole grains

If you're a bread addict, it could be tough going in the first days of your cleanse. Eliminate the cravings by switching to whole grain bread now. Increase your intake of whole grains, such as brown rice and quinoa, in favor of bread with dinner.

Switch over to healthy nondairy milk or creamers

Dairy is addictive (especially cheese) and this might be tough when you begin. Wean off dairy the week prior to your cleanse by switching to nondairy milks like hemp milk, almond milk, or coconut milk.

Eat more veggies and fruit

Now's a good time to add more seasonal vegetables and fruits to your meals and snacks. Of course, these are instead of, not in addition to, processed foods, such as cookies, chips, and crackers.

CLEANSING FOODS SHOPPING LIST

The cleansing foods listed here are for everyone, no matter what your Nutritional Style.

Vegetables, Seasonal Whenever Possible

All vegetables, except white potatoes, are on your cleanse shopping list. That includes yams and sweet potatoes. It also includes fermented vegetables, such as sauerkraut.

Fruits, Seasonal Whenever Possible

Most fruits are on the cleanse shopping list, including avocados. I particularly recommend apples, pears, blueberries, strawberries, pineapple, oranges, clementines, peaches, and seasonal fruits of all kinds. Avoid dried fruit of all kinds for now, due to the high sugar content.

Herbs, Spices, Condiments

All whole fresh or dried herbs—rosemary, tarragon, basil, thyme, oregano, etc.
All whole fresh or dried spices—turmeric, cinnamon, cumin, curry, cayenne pepper, etc.
Herbal teas for cleansing: dandelion root, milk thistle
Salt must be unprocessed sea salt
Organic vanilla or cocoa extracts

Sea Vegetables

Sea vegetables (seaweed) are a rich source of fiber, vitamins, and minerals such as iodine and magnesium. They make an excellent salt substitute. Popular sea vegetables include kombu (also called kelp), arame, nori (also called laver), hijiki, dulse, wakame, and bladderwrack. You'll probably need to buy these at your local health food store.

Beans and Legumes

All beans, including chickpeas, black beans, cannellini, pinto beans, and others. Lentils of any kind or color are also great.

Animal Protein

Most animal protein is fine while you're doing a cleanse, but it must be organic and free of hormones and antibiotics. All poultry, eggs, wild-caught fish, and red meat are good choices. Avoid pork and limit red meats to a couple of times a week.

Grains and Seeds

During your cleanse, all grains must be whole and gluten-free. Nothing made with wheat, barley, or rye should be in your diet. Good choices include brown rice, millet, oats, teff, wild rice, and quinoa.

Oils and Fats

Good fats are crucial during your cleanse. Avocados and olives are great sources of good fats. For cooking use coconut oil and grapeseed oil for high heat. Use extra virgin olive oil for low heat and salad dressings. Other choices for salad dressings are avocado oil, flaxseed oil, hemp seed oil, walnut oil, and grapeseed oil.

Nuts and Seeds

All unsalted nuts and seeds are good choices for snacks and for adding to salads and other dishes. Good seed options include hemp, chia, sunflower, and pumpkin. Nut and seed butter, such as almond butter and cashew butter, are great for sandwiches. Raw nuts and seeds are preferable to roasted to keep enzymes intact.

While all nuts are good, stay away from peanuts during your cleanse. Despite their name, peanuts are actually legumes, members of the bean family. Because they are one of the most common food allergens, peanuts aren't recommended while cleansing. Even a mild reaction to peanuts can appear as an unwanted issue in the body. Peanuts may also carry a mold called aflatoxin, which is a known carcinogen and can be toxic to the liver. Also, because peanuts have a soft shell, they're more likely to absorb toxins and pesticides from the soil. When you're done with your cleanse and want peanut butter back in your life, choose an organic brand.

Beverages

While doing the cleanse you need to drink plenty of liquids, more than you usually do. This helps flush toxins from your system as they're released. The best choice is always pure water, but you can also try these:

Nut milks: almond milk (unsweetened organic or homemade), hemp milk (unsweetened organic or homemade), any other homemade nut or seed milk (see the recipe on page 178)
Raw, pure kombucha
Freshly made vegetables juices
Freshly made fruit juices in moderation or added in small amounts to vegetable juices
Teas and herbal teas
Homemade lemonade or limeade (sweeten with stevia)

Sweeteners

Coconut sugar, liquid or crystal, in moderation
Stevia powder or liquid

Superfoods

Bee pollen to add to smoothies
Chia seeds for smoothies, salads, and to create puddings and drinks
Coconut for flavor in smoothies or stir fries
Hemp seeds to top salads and sprinkle on vegetables
Hemp protein powder for smoothies
Maca root powder for smoothies
Nutritional yeast to sprinkle on salads, popcorn, vegetables
Raw cacao nibs for smoothies
Raw cacao powder for smoothies or raw desserts

Sweets

Chocolate bars sweetened with stevia or natural sweeteners

To all you overachievers, *do not skip this key phase* in your cleanse. You won't gain anything by rushing into it. Allowing your body to adjust will ensure that you're ready, helping you to avoid uncomfortable symptoms and cravings.

Timing matters when you decide to do a cleanse. You don't need to take a month off from work, your family, and all your other responsibilities, but look ahead at your calendar when picking your start date. If you've got something major coming up over the next month—a big project deadline, business travel, or an important family event, for example—now might not be the right time. Save your cleanse for when you're not under quite so much pressure.

Remember, you're *easing* into your cleanse, and you're doing it by *adding* healthy, delicious foods that will sustain you. Add in seasonal greens and raw salads; begin to include vegetables at almost every meal. Eggs for breakfast? Sauté a quick handful of spinach alongside. Tomato sauce for the family? Try adding sliced zucchini and onion and switching over to gluten-free quinoa pasta for prep week. Lunch is always a sandwich? Switch to a salad for a few days that week.

> This cleanse is not meant to weaken you—it's meant to strengthen.

Animal Protein

Moderate amounts of animal proteins, such as chicken, turkey, beef, bison, lamb, pork, eggs, and fish, are acceptable during your cleanse if you're a Healthy Omnivore or Flexible Vegetarian. Modern Vegans on the cleanse will still rely on plant-based protein and should eliminate any yogurt or cheese in their diet.

During your prep week, cut back on your animal protein by having meatless days and by having smaller portions. This is a good way to become aware of how much animal protein you're actually eating and find ways to cut down. Begin to gather your meatless recipes and alternatives, so once cleansing begins, you can substitute *some, but not all* animal protein sources with plant-based ones. Take care not to stress your body by eliminating animal proteins too fast.

Once you begin your cleanse, it's important to listen to your body. If you begin to feel lightheaded, you may need to eat a small amount of animal protein. This cleanse is not meant to weaken you—it's meant to strengthen. Find your balance and do what feels best.

Liquid Nutrition

Each morning during your cleanse, start your day with a smoothie or, if you're a Modern Vegan, enjoy a fresh vegetable juice. Your smoothie will be loaded with a high-quality protein, fresh fruit, organic nondairy milk, such as almond or hemp milk, and some superfoods to boost your energy and your immunity. This will help you begin the day strong, with high levels of satisfying nutrients to provide sustainable energy and diminish your cravings. (Check the smoothie recipes on page 178.)

Having a liquid breakfast allows your body to awaken gently. Blending or juicing your foods assists your body by breaking down the food, liquefying it so your stomach acids don't have to, and therefore easing the digestive process. Smoothies can be a problem for people who have high blood sugar or diabetes, however. If you're unable to enjoy a smoothie or a juice because it makes your blood sugar spike, then eat a meal that is free of the foods we're eliminating, and try to add in some vegetables for fiber. For example, scrambled eggs with sautéed spinach would be an excellent cleansing alternative for Healthy Omnivores.

By adding in one liquid meal for Healthy Omnivores and Flexible Vegetarians, and at least two liquid meals for Modern Vegans (actually, if you're a Modern Vegan, you can have unlimited green juices or smoothies), you're giving your digestive system a rest by doing the work for it.

For a Healthy Omnivore, this could take some time. Begin with the creamy smoothies that contain hemp seeds or an organic plant-based protein. For Flexible Vegetarians, try a green smoothie. If you like it and it agrees with your body (no digestive upset from it), add it to your daily meal plan.

You may be afraid of the idea of a liquid breakfast, and wonder if it'll be enough to sustain you throughout the day. I've worked with elite athletes and top-level business executives who learned to start their day with a smoothie, and it's now a healthy addiction for them. Give it a try. We're discovering your personal Nutritional Style, and your cleansing style, so it's important that you feel satisfied as you begin your day. If you find a liquid breakfast isn't enough for you, add in some protein in the form of a vegetable omelet or warm quinoa with nut milk and cinnamon.

Feel completely free to adjust the quantities of your meals and experiment with the smoothie recipes included in this book or at my website. If you need to add an apple for sweetness, go ahead, unless you're sensitive to sugar.

Raw Foods

Raw vegetables, fruits, and plant-based proteins like nuts and seeds contain live enzymes, the natural proteins your body needs to break down food in your digestive tract. They're therefore often referred to as *living foods*. Heating food to above 115 degrees Fahrenheit destroys live enzymes; most cooked food therefore doesn't have any. This doesn't mean that you should never eat cooked food, because you make plenty of your own enzymes. But the more raw food you eat, the less your body needs to produce its own enzymes to digest your food. That means more energy your body can put toward other things, like making metabolic enzymes to build healthy tissues and organs, and to carry away waste. By adding in one liquid raw meal for Healthy Omnivores and Flexitarians, and at least two liquid raw meals for Modern Vegans, you're allowing your digestion to become more efficient.

All three cleansing styles will add in more raw and liquid foods for your cleanse. For Modern Vegans, a few items on your cleansing foods list need to be consumed in moderate amounts, because they are commonly cooked. Go easy on the beans, lentils, grains, and yams. The purpose of the cleanse for everyone is to add in a high percentage of raw food. If you're a Modern Vegan, you already do that. If a primarily raw diet feels too restrictive, or if you crave warmer or more substantial foods, enjoying these foods in moderation is fine.

The Nutritional Style Cleanse Protocol

OK, are you ready to begin? Let's get down to the cleanse protocols for each Nutritional Style.

THE HEALTHY OMNIVORE CLEANSE

- Liquid nutrition breakfast
- One animal protein meal a day
- Add in greens and vegetables for at least two of your meals.
- Add in whole grains, legumes, seeds, and nuts instead of additional animal protein.

Sample Menu for a Typical Day

Breakfast: creamy smoothie made with protein powder, almond milk, and fresh fruit

Lunch: fresh organic hummus and a salad loaded up with vegetables, seeds, olive oil, and lemon juice or dressing

Dinner: organic chicken breast cooked with roasted veggies and a side salad with flaxseed oil and lemon dressing

Snacks: apple, 1/4 cup almonds

If you wish, switch your animal proteins around. Have an omelet and a salad for lunch, for example, and a vegetarian chili for dinner.

THE FLEXIBLE VEGETARIAN CLEANSE

- Liquid nutrition breakfast, preferably with greens
- Alternate a day with animal protein with a day with plant-based protein only.
- Add in greens and vegetables to all your other meals.

Sample Menu for a Plant-Based Day

Breakfast: green smoothie with light and dark leafy greens and fresh fruit

Lunch: vegetable soup with brown rice and a side salad with olive oil and lemon dressing

Dinner: quinoa and bean salad with assorted field greens

Snacks: 1/2 cup blueberries or an apple, 1/4 cup nuts

Sample Menu for an Animal Protein Day

Breakfast: creamy smoothie made with organic almond or hemp milk and protein powder, fresh fruit, and superfoods such as chia seeds, flaxseeds, or maca powder.

Lunch: fresh green salad with hemp seeds, nuts, guacamole, assorted veggies and olive oil and lemon juice or a Nutritional Style dressing (several recipes are given in chapter ten).

Dinner: wild-caught salmon, sautéed broccoli and cauliflower, green salad

Snacks: 1/2 cup blueberries, or an apple, or 1/4 cup nuts

THE MODERN VEGAN CLEANSE

- Liquid nutrition for two of your three meals
- Enjoy only plant-based proteins
- Add greens and vegetables to all meals

Sample Menu for a Typical Day

Breakfast: green smoothie (see recipe in chapter ten) of blended light and dark greens, vegetables, and fruit or a green vegetable juice. You also can enjoy a more complex vegetable juice, with beets or carrots. Have enough to feel satisfied and energized.

Lunch: green smoothie, or protein smoothie made with nut or seed milk

Dinner: salad of mixed field greens and herbs with seeds, olives, nuts, vegetables, avocado, and olive oil and lemon dressing or a prepared raw food entrée, or a vegan gluten-free entrée

Snacks: green or vegetable juices or smoothies as desired, berries, apple, and nuts as desired

Tips for a Carefree Cleanse

Cleansing will be simpler and easier if you prepare not only your body but also your kitchen. Follow these tips to make it easier and more fun to stay on track with your cleanse.

Shop for your foods in advance

Having the ingredients and foods you need on hand is crucial for a successful cleanse. I want you to feel cared for during this process, and having foods on hand in the refrigerator and cupboard will allow you to feel supported. Shopping in advance and preparing your kitchen is a great way to practice taking control over your diet and your food, instead of eating whatever you find in the freezer, fridge, and pantry. Go to the market with your list and a plan, and stick to it.

Select recipes in advance

Use the recipes in this book, visit my website at HolliThompson.com for even more recipes, or explore new recipes on your own.

Carve out a preparation day or cooking day

Take a day to prepare batches of food to have on hand so that cleansing will be easier. If you have an appropriate meal waiting for

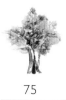

you in the fridge, you're less likely to be tempted off your cleanse. Cook up a chunky vegetable soup, a creamy asparagus soup, or a batch of vegetarian chili. Make a big batch of brown rice or quinoa, millet, or beans. Use your prep day to wash and prepare your greens for salads, and slice some carrots, onions, and kale to have on hand to sprinkle on top. Blend a raw nut pâté with vegetables to add to your luncheon salad. Use your imagination and have fun. Your cleanse is a chance to explore some new food choices and experiment with new flavors.

Eating Out in Style

I often lead group cleanses. The participants keep in touch with me and each other through a Facebook page. Brigitte posted this plea to the group: "How can we possibly eat at a restaurant while cleansing? This is going to be impossible! I'll have to stay home for two weeks!" We were just starting the cleanse, so Brigitte didn't yet know that doing a cleanse isn't an all-or-nothing proposition with a lot of deprivation. I quickly responded to Brigitte and the group by telling them that you can eat out almost anywhere, even while doing a cleanse, and still maintain your Nutritional Style.

Here are my best tips for dining out, now and forever:

Ask for a big glass of water as soon as you're seated. Drinking water cuts your hunger, hydrates you after a long day, and gives you some energy. It'll also fortify you for making good decisions. You'll be able to peruse the menu without going crazy while calmly enjoying the company of your fellow diners.

While cleansing, skip the wine or other alcohol. Instead, order sparkling mineral water with some lime or lemon. You've got this. Just think how good you'll feel in the morning. After your cleanse, a wine spritzer is a good option. If an expensive fine wine is on the table, have just one glass instead.

Ask the waiter to remove the bread basket, or at least put it out of arm's reach. You don't want to stare at the house special rolls as they taunt you from the center of the table. Ask your waiter to please remove them. If your date or other diners are digging in, nudge the basket across the table, out of reach.

Order salad as an appetizer, always. You can never overdo your raw greens, so take advantage of fresh greens while you're out. If you can get your salad with some nuts, go for it. Ask for vinaigrette dressing on the side.

If you're a Healthy Omnivore, order fresh fish. Because most nice restaurants have daily fish deliveries, this is a good time to enjoy seafood, if you eat it. Ask for it baked, grilled, or lightly sautéed in olive oil. Say no to creamy sauces. (Hate seafood? Try the chicken.)

If you're a Flexible Vegetarian or Modern Vegan, discuss your preferences with your waiter. Today many restaurants offer a choice of yummy vegetarian and vegan dishes that are real food, not afterthoughts on the menu. Ditto for gluten-free dishes. Many chefs are also willing to modify a dish on the menu to accommodate vegetarians and vegans. At worst, you can always ask your waiter for a big salad or a platter of vegetables, and maybe some whole grains if they're available.

Take care of your digestion. You don't want this meal out to bloat your belly (that dress is way too chic!), so practice food combining. If you're having grains for dinner, skip the animal protein. If you're having animal protein, skip the grains. Order a double vegetable side instead. Like this: Ordering chicken or fish? Skip the side rice and double up on the broccoli. Craving the whole-grain pasta? Enjoy it with a simple vegetable marinara. This will make your dinner easier to digest and you'll still look svelte when you stand up.

Skip dessert. You should be completely full and satisfied after this meal, so order an herbal tea and relax. That sly smile says it all. You just ate out while cleansing!

What to Expect During Your Cleanse

Cleansing is an energizing experience, but it's also a detoxifying process. That means you should expect some changes as your body lets go of toxins and they make their way out of your system. As you work through the cleanse, early detoxification signs, like headaches, weakness and fatigue, or achy joints, indicate that the cleanse is working—you're feeling the effects of the toxins being eliminated from your diet. This is normal, even desirable, but if it's becoming difficult to make it through the day, slow down. Fatigue is often related to not drinking enough. Make sure you're drinking enough pure water each day—aim for at least six glasses. If you're feeling tired, make allowances for it. Give yourself more rest time during the day and get to bed earlier at night. It may seem counterintuitive, but adding in some gentle exercise for half an hour a day can actually help counter fatigue and achiness by boosting your energy and getting your blood circulating. If you can, enjoy a sauna or warm bath several times a week while you detox. The heat is relaxing and helps draw toxins out through your skin. Adding a handful of Epsom salts to your bath is recommended, for both relaxation as well as detoxification benefits.

Regular elimination is important as you cleanse, so make sure that you're having a bowel movement at least once a day. You may start to feel backed up—this can happen at first as your body gets used to the higher level of fiber you take in during a cleanse. If you do, an old-fashioned enema using warm water may be very helpful to gently ease toxins from your body. I don't recommend packaged enemas; they contain unwanted chemicals. You can also explore having a colonic. Be very selective when you look for a colonic practitioner. Although colonics are generally very safe, this is an unregulated area. Get strong recommendations before making the appointments.

On the positive side, after the first few days most people begin to feel increased energy and their thinking becomes more clear. Your

ERIN The Cleanse that Didn't Work

Erin signed up for a group cleanse with me. During the first week, she attended a Q&A phone conference that I hosted for all participants. She complained on the call that she was feeling quite sick. Given the gentleness of the cleanse she was doing, I thought it couldn't be the cleanse itself that was making her feel ill; perhaps Erin had a virus or the flu. Her symptoms were beyond any normal reaction I'd ever seen.

I asked about her foods and daily routine. When she got to the part where she talked about her cleanse supplements, I didn't recognize them as anything I'd ever recommended. It turns out that Erin had heard about a new cleanse kit with herbal supplements from one of her fellow moms. She had decided to take them along with the work we were doing together. It was all too much for her body.

She was sick as a dog, and justifiably so. I explained that the cleanse was carefully planned out and that it wasn't a good idea to add in another protocol. We got rid of those supplements, pronto, and stopped the cleanse. A few days later, Erin said she was feeling a lot better. We agreed that she should wait a couple of weeks and then try the cleanse again, without adding anything beyond the protocol. This time, Erin did a lot better and completed the cleanse without any trouble.

I now make sure to add that piece to my instructions. Don't double up your cleanse protocol!

mood lifts, and you feel happier, often for no reason in particular. When you look in the mirror, your skin looks clear and younger. Bonus! Your eyes look clearer, too, and puffiness and signs of aging seem to gently fade.

If you do feel some unpleasant side effects don't be fooled into thinking the healthy food on your cleanse is what makes you feel that way. Some mild discomfort is expected; it doesn't mean you aren't meant to live a healthy lifestyle. It just means you might be detoxing too fast and it's time to be more gradual with your efforts.

Easing Off Your Cleanse

Congratulations! You've finished the two weeks of the cleanse—or you tried your best to complete it. It's hard to change your eating habits, and even though your common sense may desire change, I realize how tough it can be. You get kudos from me just for making the effort. Now it's time to gradually ease back into your preferred Nutritional Style eating approach. Over the next week or so, slowly

DANA Cleanse Success

Dana came to me for a private consultation to get help for her gastroesophageal reflux (GERD) symptoms. In addition to the discomfort from her severe heartburn, Dana got sick frequently, and was experiencing some autoimmune issues as well.

Dana had never explored food intolerances as a root cause to any of her symptoms. Despite her GERD and her frequent illnesses, she believed she was eating a healthy diet. In fact, as I explained to her, Dana was eating a lot of inflammatory foods every day. They were probably the main reason her GERD symptoms were so frequent and painful.

After going through her health history, I recommended that Dana do a cleanse. She enthusiastically agreed, seeing it as a chance to jump-start some changes she hoped would help the GERD symptoms. Almost immediately after starting the cleanse,

Dana felt a lot better. This was a bit surprising to me, because most people take longer to feel the benefits, but clearly Dana's symptoms were triggered by gluten, dairy, and sugar. Once we took these out of her diet, her reflux practically disappeared and she began to feel more energetic. By the time Dana finished her cleanse, she felt like a new person; a completely improved version of herself.

By eating a diet better suited to her Nutritional Style, Dana was feeling good, knowing that she'd taken significant steps toward taking charge of her own health. After her cleanse, Dana signed on with me to learn more. She began to make smoothies each day, bought a high-speed blender, and her previously reluctant husband joined her on her new path. Dana is a new person who now rarely gets sick. We're hoping that her health issues are far behind her!

start to add in more of your usual foods. What I hope you've gained from the cleanse is a new appreciation of the value of vegetables. Don't be surprised if you find that you continue to crave them once the cleanse is over. This is one craving I definitely encourage!

Don't be self-critical if you pooped out early. Some of my clients find that after they complete the prep week, they realize how far they still have to go. They feel they're not ready yet for a full cleanse. That's fine—the important thing is that they're moving forward with increased awareness. If that's you, excellent! Transforming your eating style takes time. I remember when I first changed my diet, and how difficult it was.

Improvements in your diet and health are a process. You're in it for the long haul, not just for the four weeks of a cleanse. Keep going, and see what else is in store. Keep trying new recipes, and varying your ingredients to find the combinations that satisfy you and keep your energy high. You can come back to cleansing when you're ready.

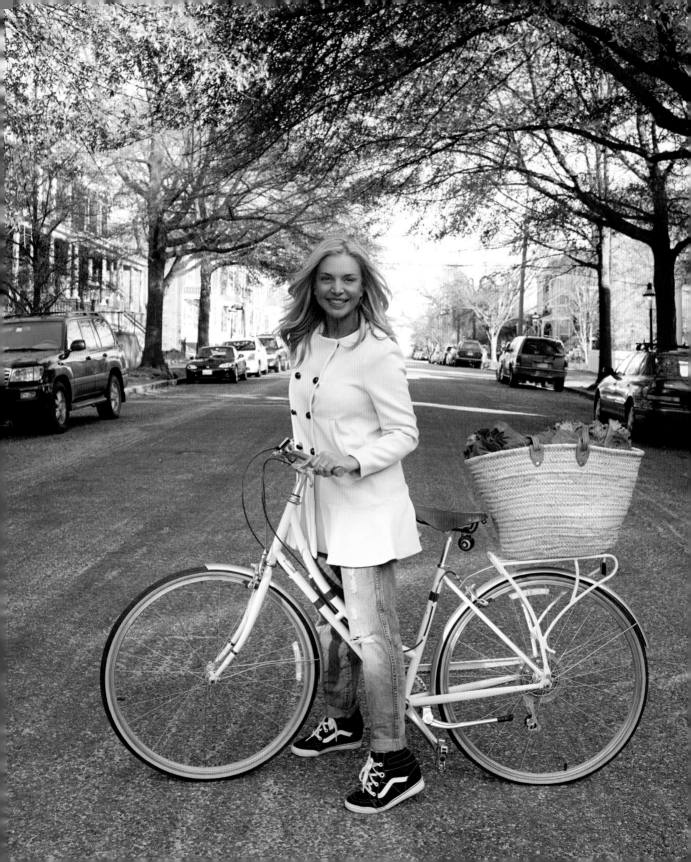

CHAPTER FIVE

Healing in Style

My sister Jackie was diagnosed with breast cancer in 2002. Thankfully, she responded well to treatment. Today she's healthy and hasn't had a recurrence. She never told us how advanced her cancer was. Looking back, I realize that was her way of not creating more concern than the family already felt. It would only serve to label her and worry us more.

I felt completely unprepared and scared to deal with anyone who had cancer, much less my own big sister. I was the little sister who became completely incompetent when faced with the big C. Actually, I wasn't the only one. We hadn't yet faced anything like this as a family, and it was hard for everyone—except, apparently, Jackie. We took turns going along with her to her chemotherapy sessions. When my turn came, I was nervous about it, sure that it was a horrible and scary process. Jackie was a bit surprised that we all wanted to go along. She basically said, "Well, come if you want, but it's not a big deal. Why does everyone want to take me to chemo?"

What else could we possibly do?

At her chemo session, I was invisible, despite all my effort and concern. Jackie chatted with strangers and patients. She talked to everyone there that day. She asked the other women how they felt, shared where she bought her latest wig, and was supportive to everyone receiving treatment. I wondered when my oldest sister had become Florence Nightingale and why she had never gone into nursing.

My sister had told me about the lump in her breast earlier that year, during a visit she and her husband made to our farm. She told me she had a tiny lump, which she had found herself, and that it hadn't shown up when she went for a mammogram. Her

It often takes something scary, a life-or-death scenario, to make people go for serious changes in their diet and lifestyle.

doctor told her not to worry—just recheck it in a few months. I was concerned and suggested that she shouldn't wait. She ended up having surgery just a couple of weeks later.

Because her cancer was estrogen-sensitive, Jackie realized that she now needed to avoid soy foods, which can mimic estrogen in the body. She immediately went through her pantry. She threw out boxes of her favorite breakfast cereal, the one she's been eating almost every day for years, because it contained highly processed soy. She had chosen the brand because the box proclaimed it was a healthy choice. She tore through her cupboards and got rid of all the processed and refined foods. Fortunately, she and her husband are both great cooks, so the decision to switch to a diet of whole foods prepared at home wasn't hard, at least from the cooking end. The buying end was more difficult. She would call me from the super-market to say that everything she was looking at had processed soy, added sugar, or both. She described the grocery store as a carnival, with processed food packages screaming, "Buy me! Buy me!"

When I became a health coach, Jackie was my first client. I was skeptical that this new relationship would work. After all, in my training I'd been cautioned not to work with family members, because they often don't listen to those closest to them. But she proved to be a star client. She embraced her new foods, fitness, and overall healthy lifestyle with grace and enthusiasm. In fact, she became as passionate as I was about her personal health.

Then, just a few years ago, my sister Lea was diagnosed with lung cancer. Although she had smoked for part of her adult life, her cancer was found to be from environmental causes, not tobacco. If there's a good kind of lung cancer to have, this was it. Her progno-sis was, and is, excellent. In fact, after surgery she didn't need any further treatment. Lea also changed her approach to her diet after her cancer, switching to more organic foods and eating in an over-all healthier way. Yes, she bought a juicer immediately, but she also tweaked her overall diet and lifestyle. She and her husband removed all harmful chemicals from their environment. They began using safer cleaning products, soaps, and skin care products. They even started using organic pest removal (see Lea's solution for ants in her home on page 123). When I visited their home in Florida, I was sur-prised and so happy to find my lovely sister thriving, and with a new awareness of environmental toxins.

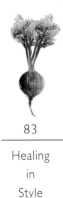

It often takes something scary, a life-or-death scenario, to make people go for serious changes in their diet and lifestyle. Cancer does it for many people. Most people go through life hoping for the best, and thinking that their bodies will be able to handle the toxic chemicals that they come into contact with each day. They roll the dice on their health, even when they know they're intolerant to gluten, or dairy, or sugar. When a health crisis does happen, they don't want to make the conscious leap from their diet and lifestyle to their disease. They don't understand that eating whatever it is will create inflammation, and that year after year of chronic inflammation can cause a wide range of health problems. And yes, maybe even the big C.

In 2011, I met a prominent oncology surgeon at a hunt breakfast in Middleburg, Virginia. Dr. Eleni Tousimis was living and practicing in New York City at the time. We connected quickly on many things, but especially on the importance of food in healing. When Dr. Tousimis took a new job in Washington, D.C., as director of the breast health program at Georgetown University Hospital, she called me. She asked if she could refer recently diagnosed breast cancer patients to me for help with their food and nutrition. She wanted me to do something special for these women—most of them were still reeling from the news of a cancer diagnosis. Thinking of my sisters, I responded, "Of course." Then I asked if there was anything specific she wanted me to tell them. Her response was, "Just teach them how to eat well. Most of them don't really know what healthy eating is. They only think they do. They could use some help." OK, I thought, this will be a real challenge. Before I felt ready to begin, I did a lot of background research into the science supporting a connection between a good diet and cancer prevention, especially the prevention of breast cancer recurrences.

My first client, Heather, was a successful art dealer who traveled a lot on business; she was married and had two children. To her, breast cancer was just an inconvenient addition to her busy life. She was sure that her diet was already healthy enough. After all, she told me, she ate a salad each day at lunch. She was shaken by her cancer diagnosis, though, and with her husband sitting by her side, we had our first conversation. She wanted to do everything possible to help her heal from surgery, support her body through chemo, and allow her to live a healthy life. She wanted to see her children grow up.

We worked through her diet together and found that she needed more calories, particularly calories from protein. Then we started to

> Just teach them how to eat well. Most of them don't really know what healthy eating is.

add in healthy foods—superfoods, smoothies, pressed juices, and salads with lots of dark green leafy veggies, not the plain romaine lettuce she used to eat. Heather ordered a Vitamix and a home juicer. More important, she made time in her busy life for self-care, starting with taking the time to eat a more varied diet and to choose better foods. We made shopping lists and menu plans. We took a walk around the neighborhood of her art gallery. We found all the local shops and cafes that offered quality food she could grab for a quick lunch.

Because she was a popular social figure, her friends and colleagues all wanted to help. How do we help? With food, of course. People were constantly stopping by her gallery or home, bearing cheesy casseroles, lasagna, and cookies. We created a "foods allowed" list for Heather, and we asked all of her well-meaning circle of friends to comply. We posted a superfoods list on her personal website so that those who wanted to help could contribute edibles she really needed to eat. We didn't compromise just to be polite, which was difficult for Heather at first. As it turned out, yes, a few people were offended; everyone else went along, with minimal grumbling.

Heather decided she wanted to give up animal protein. I worked with her to ensure that her diet would be a healthy vegan diet, with enough protein for healing. Even vegans can end up eating manufactured foods laced with chemicals, though, so I also taught Heather how to read food labels and choose unprocessed, whole foods whenever possible.

She dove into this new way of eating like a champion, embracing it enthusiastically and with a smile. Our next step was to remove all processed foods. Eventually we worked up to removing gluten, sugar, and dairy, foods that can create an inflammatory reaction. She didn't falter. We worked together over five months, continuously tweaking her diet. Just as important, I supported Heather in her choice to pursue a healthier lifestyle. Change is hard—we all need help.

Heather had a long road ahead of her, but she got through it without any serious difficulty. She was able to eat well even when she was nauseous and fatigued from chemotherapy. She's still in treatment, but she feels good and her outlook has remained positive. Most of all, she has the energy she wants and needs. She told me that her doctors were thrilled with her progress, and that she has never felt better. Looking back, Heather gives a great deal of credit to her healthy eating.

> Change is hard—
> we all need help.

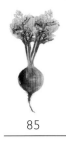

Since then I've worked with many women to help them move beyond their cancer diagnosis, get through treatment, and come out the other side. I love these women. They're optimistic, determined, and happy in their lives. Their diagnosis doesn't define them. They just want to get better and never have to deal with this again. They know in their hearts that there's a connection between what we put in our mouths and our health. When faced with cancer, they want to make big changes, now.

We go for it. I work with them by phone (easiest for everyone, especially these successful DC and NYC women) or in person. They're ready for change and they are the best clients, ever.

We start by dissecting their diet. Everyone has something to tweak, and these women are motivated beyond anyone else. We work through their day, meal by meal. While I usually begin with adding in more healthy foods, with cancer patients we speak simultaneously about what to remove as well.

We add a rainbow of colorful vegetables full of phytonutrients. I encourage them to eat cruciferous vegetables, such as broccoli, cabbage, brussels sprouts, and turnips. These foods contain, among many other beneficial compounds, something called glucosinolates, which may have valuable anticancer effects in humans. Ditto for leafy greens, such as kale, arugula, mustard greens, and collards. I help them select a juicer and teach them how to use it; I send them to their local organic juice bar. I encourage them to eat seasonally and locally, if possible.

I recommend superfoods like chia seeds and hemp seeds for their morning smoothie. These seeds are a great source of omega-3 fatty acids, which are essential to our health and maintaining a good balance of anti-inflammatory hormones. We add more cancer-fighting phytonutrients from green leafy veggies to the smoothie to start their day in a balanced and supportive way. I give them recipes and ideas for smoothies that will suit them and their taste buds, and we make sure that it all tastes delicious. Sometimes cancer treatment can mess with the sense of taste. Some patients find that foods they normally love don't taste very good anymore. Because it's important to get enough calories even when your food tastes lousy, I work with them to find the foods they can still enjoy. One of my clients craved oranges; there was something about the fresh sweetness that tasted incredibly delicious to her after chemo treatment. Others crave salty foods—everyone is different. During this difficult time, I tell my clients that if they hate the way something tastes, even if it's good for them, why eat it? Go instead for something that you love and that still tastes good—just try to stay within the overall boundaries.

And then we remove things, like processed and refined foods stripped of their natural nutrients and filled with chemicals and additives. We take away inflammatory foods. I often start my clients off with a gentle cleanse, using whole foods, to help them tune into their bodies and discover if they do, indeed, have any food intolerances. Especially at a time when your body is under a lot of stress, it's important to learn about and avoid any intolerances.

I also ask my clients to limit alcohol or avoid it altogether. Any positive effects of drinking red wine, for instance, are outweighed by the high sugar content and the inflammatory response that alcohol can create. Alcohol can remove inhibitions, and for many, this can create cravings and cause overeating. Best to stay away, with just the occasional glass of wine.

Along with dietary changes, I insist that my clients move. It's non-negotiable. Many, many scientific studies show the positive effect of exercise in general for cancer prevention. Many scientific studies also confirm that regular exercise can help prevent recurrence in breast cancer patients. I ask my clients to invest in a new pair of kicks or yoga socks, please. A healthy weight after breast cancer is another key factor in preventing recurrence, according to numerous studies. For my clients, that's a great incentive for weight loss, and their new lifestyle helps them along.

When you remove the junk, add in the good stuff and begin to exercise, the resulting effects are not only physical, but mental and emotional as well. Improved clarity of thought, less fatigue, and better moods are common side effects. And if you're in a happier place, with a brighter outlook, that helps your overall health by strengthening your immunity. A stronger, healthier immunity means—you got it—more power to fight off a recurrence and disease of any kind.

Don't wait for the cancer diagnosis. Don't roll those dice. Take control of your health now by following the steps outlined in this book. Move toward a simple, sound approach that works.

> When you remove the junk, add in the good stuff and begin to exercise.

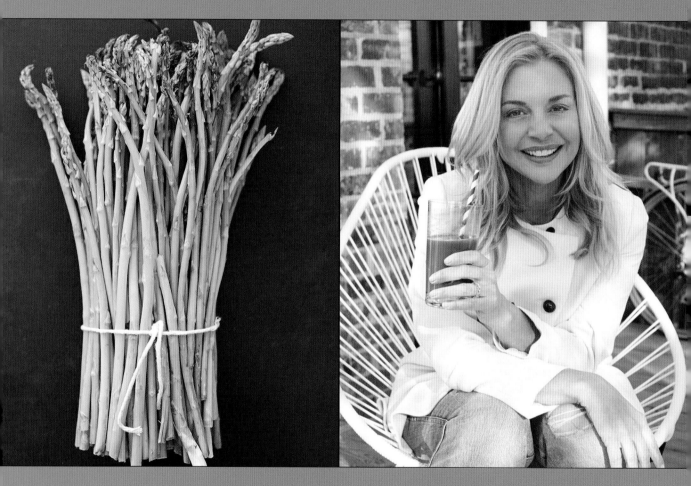

Because we are all part of nature,
we each feel the energy of the seasons.

CHAPTER SIX

Enter Spring

Spring: there's something new and sexy in the air, a feeling that anything is possible, a feeling that—like the plants, trees, and flowers—you can be reborn. Whether in a garden, a park, or strolling down Fifth Avenue in the middle of Manhattan, you feel the soft energy that spring brings. Where I live, near Washington, DC, the scenery gradually turns from faded brown to a soft, vibrant green. Later, it becomes dotted with the pinks and delicate whites of early-blossoming cherry trees that blow petals across the sidewalks for a precious few days. Vibrant tulips stand tall and gorgeous, and daffodils shine their yellow petals, sometimes emerging from early-spring snow.

Your body wants to wake up, move, and get outside to soak up the soft, hazy sunshine of April and May. You feel an irresistible desire to turn your face upward toward the sun, just like the daffodils, and breathe deeply.

Springtime feels like a reward for suffering through the long, cold winter. With the plentiful, gentle spring rains come warmer weather and a lighter feeling as you shed the heavy layers of winter covering. Working at home all winter, I tend to get into a rut about what I wear. Each year, as spring comes I feel the urge to burn my black fleece jackets and yoga pants and add color to my wardrobe. I crave pink and peach and gorgeous blues, lighter nail polish, and nude-colored sandals. I leave the black suede pumps and bags behind and reach for vibrant hues, even in my running shoes or yoga clothes. My husband pulls out his polos and shorts, and even if the temperature dips a little, we're ready for warm weather.

Spring brings new energy to life, with longer, lighter days and seemingly more time on your hands. It's no longer pitch black before 5:00 p.m., and if you're like me, you once again are drawn to impromptu dinners out, a late walk, the gym, or a yoga class. You have more energy late in the day, and you feel the urge to get out and use it, rather than crashing on the sofa.

This is the time for spring-cleaning of all kinds. On the first warm days, you air out your home and throw open the windows—the whole house feels fresh and new. You shake out the kitchen rugs, clean the windowsills, sweep off the porch, and dust off the clay herb pots. You consider repainting the front door and planting annual flowers, and start thinking about mowing the lawn.

Because we are all part of nature, we each feel the energy of the seasons; the dormant energy of winter has given way to a fresh life force bursting all around. As the trees get ready to blossom and the new flowers peek up through the snow, you're feel the same energy and resurgence of life. On a cellular level, you're programmed to lighten your foods and get active again.

This can bring some unwelcome pressure—as you peel away bulky winter layers, you may not yet feel ready for your close up. While the rest of the world is having fun, dining al fresco at sidewalk cafés or running in the park, you might be disappointed to discover that you gained some pounds over the winter; your running shorts are now too tight to fit over your hips. You've spent the winter on the sofa or behind a desk, and now everyone around you is moving faster—jogging, running, walking—while you feel like you're in quicksand.

You need solutions, and you need them now.

Spring Clean Your Diet

As I explained back in chapter four, a nutritional cleanse in the spring is part of the natural way of life. It helps you transition physically and mentally from the quiet of winter into the active style of the new season. Notice the foods you naturally choose in spring. For an Easter brunch, you want baby root vegetables, asparagus, and tender greens—all are high in fiber and beneficial to your digestion. A cleanse in spring should be gentle and easy, because spring is naturally the time of year for lighter, easy-to-digest, cleansing foods. No one would serve a hearty beef stew at a dinner party during the warm days of May. You'd probably make something lighter, like fresh wild salmon, or switch out a heavy bean stew for quinoa with loads of fresh veggies and seasonal leafy greens.

The baby vegetables of spring—radishes, carrots, and baby beets—are small and tender and therefore easier to digest than the later harvest of the fall. The spring harvest is traditionally simple and spare. Fruits are not plentiful yet, and early berries are light and delicate.

Historically, in the days before refrigeration and freezers, our eating patterns naturally adjusted with the seasons. Our food choices reflected what was available because there were no other options. Frozen vegetables, fruits, and meats only became available to consumers in the 1930s. By the 1950s, the TV dinner had been invented and canned, frozen, and processed convenience foods became widely available. Most homemakers were thrilled to have the luxury of a wide array of choices for preparing their families' meals. Feeding the family became simpler. Moms could serve their children green beans from a can any time of year and pour peaches drenched in sweet syrup over store-bought cakes. When Mom was ready for a night off, she could pop a TV dinner in the oven and serve it in minutes. Life was good, or so they thought.

My husband's mother was an accomplished woman and a devoted minister for a church in New England at a time when most mothers were wearing aprons and not part of the workforce. According to my husband, his family's meals were filled with canned vegetables, boxed cake mixes, and frozen dinners. He still jokes about how he never knew what a fresh green bean looked like until he was twenty-five. Both of my in-laws were enthusiastic about these new convenience foods. My husband's parents considered it a luxury not to have to prepare foods from scratch. To my father-in-law, a busy, working immigrant from Norway, this was part of the American dream.

In contrast to my husband's Wonder Bread upbringing, my childhood was all about eating unprocessed foods in season. My parents were, and still are, whole foodies. My mother turned her nose up at anything frozen, and refused to buy me blueberries flown in from Chile when I saw them at the supermarket in February. She told me my favorite fruit was out of season, not freshly picked, and full of pesticides. Despite my longing, I would have to wait.

My parents treated grocery shopping as a sport or some kind of contest, negotiating over the ripeness of each cantaloupe, smelling tomatoes, reaching for only the freshest locally grown lettuces. It was their quality time together. Boxed cake mixes were unwelcome in our home. My mother made cakes and pies from scratch, even after packaged versions' popularity soared.

She was a food adventurer. When my part-English, part-Swedish mother married my father, a first-generation American of Italian descent, she quickly integrated his mother's recipes from central

> On a cellular level, you're programmed to lighten your foods and get active again.

SPRING SUPERFOODS

The first tender produce of the spring is a tantalizing hint of the vegetable abundance soon to come. Now's the time to enjoy baby greens, mini carrots, crispy radishes, early spinach—and to experiment with other spring superfoods. Check out this list of the best superfoods of the season:

Artichokes

Artichokes are my family's favorite food. This springtime gem is a good source of calcium, folate, dietary fiber, and vitamins C and K. Artichokes are packed with antioxidants and if eaten whole, leaf by leaf, take a long time to enjoy—a bonus for practicing slower, mindful eating. Look for firm, dark green, and unblemished globes. Any good vegetarian cookbook will explain how to prepare and trim them to cook. My guys love them steamed and served with a simple vinaigrette dipping sauce or melted (organic, grass-fed) butter.

Asparagus

This tender veggie always reminds me of spring; its delicate taste and limited harvest make it all the more desirable. Asparagus is a good source of iron, fiber, and vitamins A, C, E, and K. It also contains folate, which works along with vitamin B12 to prevent mental decline. Who knew? Asparagus for anti-aging! I like the diuretic properties of asparagus as well—it's a good way to remove swelling and bloat.

Strawberries

When the first strawberries appear on our farm, we know summer's not far off. My son and I used to pick them together when he was young; they're tiny and sweet and I can still picture his smiling little face stained with red berry juice. A great source of potassium and vitamin C, strawberries are a delicious way to strengthen your immunity, repair your skin, and add a touch of sweet to your springtime smoothie.

Italy, using handpicked vegetables and beans from the garden. My sisters and I used to beg for frozen TV dinners, which we thought were fun and cool, but we were allowed to have them only on rare occasions.

My family's eating style was radically different from my friends' families. My mother branched into continental cuisine long before it became popular. My friends gazed in wonder at the exotic meals she served them when they stayed at our house for dinner. Many of her offerings they had never seen before, like Greek moussaka, stuffed artichokes, bean and Swiss chard soup, and sweetbreads sautéed in lemon and garlic.

Meanwhile, the rest of the developed world grabbed hold of convenience foods, enjoying their ease and extended shelf life. Fast food restaurants multiplied, providing quick, low-cost family meals.

No country dove in to the world of convenience food with as

Spring onions

Also known as scallions or green onions, spring onions are actually baby onions that haven't yet grown into a full bulb. Containing vitamins A, B, C, and K, spring onions are rich in minerals, such as calcium, and provide anti-inflammatory benefits. Like other members of the allium family, including garlic, leeks, and chives, spring onions help to fight viruses, making them a perfect choice to fend off spring colds.

Radishes

I love baby radishes fresh from the farm in spring, sprinkled with Himalayan sea salt and nothing else. As members of the cruciferous family of veggies, along with broccoli and cabbage, radishes offer powerful antioxidants and cancer-fighting benefits. They're a good source of magnesium and vitamin C. Their spicy and cooling flavor is also said to break down mucus, the springtime solution to your winter cold. You can prepare and enjoy large varieties, like black or watermelon radishes, as you would any other root vegetable—in soups, stews, or roasted in the oven. Daikon radish is popular in Ayurvedic medicine, where it's used to promote digestion and detoxification.

Leafy greens, especially arugula, spinach, and salad greens

After a long winter, the first spring greens are a real pleasure. They taste best at this time of year: tender, delicate, and flavorful. Greens are cleansing to the body, plus they're a great source of beta carotene (your body converts this to vitamin A), vitamin K, calcium, and potassium. Enjoying the abundance of leafy greens in spring helps to detox the heavy foods of winter and provides an energy boost, too. Enjoy leafy greens in lots of ways: juice them, use them in smoothies and salads, or sauté them—salad greens are delicious when they're lightly cooked. Try cutting a romaine lettuce in half vertically and putting the pieces on the grill for a few minutes. Drizzle with extra-virgin olive oil, lemon, and sea salt for a savory new way to enjoy your greens.

much gusto as did the United States. In the 1950s, it was hard to see where this would lead, but by end of the century, easy, fast, cheap food fed a nation of overweight, unhealthy people.

Today, the United States especially, and increasingly other countries, face a continuing rise in obesity, diabetes, heart disease, and cancer. We're now mired in a health crisis of proportions we've never seen before, partly because of the widespread availability of chemically altered and processed foods.

Created in factories, processed foods contain ingredients that sound more like supplies for a chemistry experiment than food. Sadly, the processed foods of my husband's childhood seem almost healthy compared to today's increasingly toxic versions. Convenience food companies use cheap manufactured ingredients (many genetically modified) and grossly undertested chemical additives, resulting in food that in my opinion no longer qualifies as food.

Shed Your Winter Self

As explained in chapter four, a spring cleanse is a great opportunity to rid your body of the effects these artificial ingredients leave behind. The natural cleansing qualities of spring that, by design, once naturally assisted the body's transition from winter, today require your conscious attention. Because of the intrusions of modern life, your body now needs assistance to remove the foreign chemicals that it doesn't recognize or want. As the great comedian Robin Williams says, "Spring is nature's way of saying, 'Let's party!'"

Start the party with a cleanse, and keep it going by adding exercise to your life. Spring is a time for new activity, and even if you're not planting a field or mulching your garden, you still feel it. It's like a new day, a new beginning. Even if you hate gardening, you have seeds to plant in the metaphorical sense. Your body and your mind are programmed to get busy at this time of year, so whatever it is you feel called to do, listen. Now is the time to move.

> Even if you hate gardening, you have seeds to plant in the metaphorical sense.

Much as you know that exercise and movement are essential to your health, you still might not be doing much or any moving. Maybe you've gone through times when you've hit your fitness groove and you know what it feels like to be toned and sleek and sweaty. You know the endorphin rush that's possible when you raise your heart rate for a sustained period. Maybe you know the feeling of being naturally energized after a long bike ride, or the exaltation of climbing a mountain to enjoy a view that inspires you beyond belief.

Perhaps it's the increased metabolism and fat burn that you crave from being fit, and knowing that you actually have to eat foods to support you and your sporty activities, to get the energy you need to perform well.

On the other hand, you might be a permanent fixture at your desk, kitchen table, or on your wraparound sofa. Exercise for you is fluffing pillows, walking to the mailbox, or running out for a latte. Maybe exercise is *your* personal challenge in finding the healthiest you possible.

I've learned that if I don't move and add some form of exercise to my day, everything gets more difficult. Maybe I should reframe that.

If I exercise, and move regularly, everything gets easier. My brain works better and my creativity improves. (Some of my best blog posts have come after a breathless run or a fun, sporty day.) My weight stabilizes, and if I do need to drop a few pounds, exercise is a key ingredient that helps the fat melt away.

You might not be an exercise fan. You might hate the idea of sweating, think you don't have time for the gym, or live in an urban area where walking means dodging other pedestrians and cars. Believe me, my clients have given me a lot of excuses, often good ones, for their lack of exercise. Do it anyway. You know in your heart that I'm right. You know you'd feel amazing if you exercised every day, or heck, every other day, or even every few days. Exercising for just 10 minutes a day every few days might be a huge accomplishment for you—and that would be an excellent start.

Experts tell us that all you need for a big improvement in fitness and health is 30 minutes of activity most days. You don't have to pay for gym membership or find a yoga studio. Just walk for half an hour. If you can't do that, ride an exercise bike or do a simple workout with light weights while watching TV. It makes the guilty pleasure of watching mindless TV seem a little more worthwhile.

I challenge you to move, starting today, to be able to say you're doing something for your body and that *it feels really good.* Start gently, and slowly; you don't have to compete with anyone.

Walk Out the Door

When I first began health coaching, I quickly became busy with new clients. It was wonderful and rewarding, but my enthusiasm took over, and my fitness program took a nosedive.

After a couple of months of moving only on weekends, I knew I needed to walk my own talk, and I became determined to change my exercise patterns. If I had been working in my office, I'd walk down the road and back, sometimes just for 20 minutes if that was all I could spare. If I had to drive into town, I'd take 10 minutes to walk around and window shop.

I coach my clients who work in the city to walk out of their office buildings and go pick up their own lunch from the healthy place that's five blocks away. Even the shortest walk can be beneficial to your body and mind. As you go through your day, look for opportunities to add in some steps. Take the stairs instead of the elevator,

Resent having to exercise? Walk. It's free, you already know how to do it, and you can do it anywhere. Some tips to get you going:

1. Add some tunes.

Adding music can inspire you to move and uplift your spirits, and might even encourage a real-life "happy dance." Load up your iPod or phone with your favorite tunes and get back to that music lovin' person you used to be.

2. Do what you can.

You don't have to walk two or three miles to get benefits. Just a quick 20-minute session can improve your fitness level and put a smile on your face.

3. Walking to and from counts.

Add walking into your day any way you can. That might mean walking to and from the office, or walking to pick up take-out lunch or dinner, or parking far away from the entrance to your favorite department store.

4. No sneakers required.

If you can keep a pair of sneakers in your desk drawer, tote, or car, so much the better, but you can walk in any shoes (OK, not the Jimmy Choos). Slip on some low, comfortable shoes, or if you're near soft grass or sand, go barefoot.

5. Find other ways to add steps.

Doing housework, weeding the garden, walking the dog—they're all good exercise. Just try to make the activity last for at least 20 minutes nonstop.

walk down the hall to see a colleague rather than calling, take a walk break rather than a coffee break, get off the bus a stop earlier, walk your kid to school.

The human body is not meant to sit around all day, and a sedentary lifestyle might actually be one of the worst things you can do for your health—mental and physical. In fact, recent research suggests that people who sit more than four hours a day, even if they also get regular exercise, die sooner than people who do less sitting.

One of my clients and a dear friend, Lisa, is a great example of keeping fit. If she needs to move, she'll literally walk out her door and return 45 minutes later. She doesn't feel the need to change into Lycra leggings or even running shoes. She just does it. She walks out the door, down the hill, and gets her heart rate up. She'll jump on her kid's bike and ride down the road, just like when she was a girl. She wears whatever walking shoes she has on, or she steps barefoot onto the grass.

We were like that as kids. We jumped on our bikes or walked a mile or more to see a friend and play. Lisa still does it, and she's been "naturally" thin her entire adult life. Other women think she must have a fast metabolism, or that she eats like a bird, but neither is true. She lives the "just do it" philosophy, and she knows her body. If it's time to move, she does.

Your Springtime Skin

When you finally take off those winter leggings, do you shriek in horror at the scales on your skin that have emerged over the winter? Hello, alligator legs! Maybe you're scratching and feeling itchy from months of wearing wool, and your skin longs to feel smooth and soft again.

The skin is the body's largest organ, and it's part of the system for eliminating toxins. You shed approximately a million skin cells a day, a statistic that made me wonder, where does it go? Then I learned that they collect in your house as "dust." Maybe you'd rather not know that.

If your skin is dry and rough, you might want to help your body to speed the process that allows new skin cells to emerge sooner, and reclaim that baby-soft skin. Let's explore some easy, natural ways to get sleek skin in time for summer, for both your body and your face.

Revealing a more beautiful you

Dry brushing your skin is an ancient exfoliation method. It's easy, inexpensive, and highly effective, a trifecta of virtues. I've had people write me to thank me for this simple tip. A sample:

> Dear Holli,
> I loved doing the cleanse with you, but I wanted to tell you
> that the simple tip about dry brushing has changed my life.
> Just as you said, it felt funny at first, but my skin is now
> soft and smooth. For me, that's a miracle. I've had rough
> skin most of my adult life. Thank you for this easy, but
> fabulous, tip!

Exfoliate in Latin means "to strip of leaves," and many cultures have historically practiced dry brushing or some other form of natural exfoliation. Dry skin brushing works to gently remove dead skin cells, aids in stimulating circulation, assists the lymphatic system in removing toxins from the body, and promotes healthy, glowing skin. It's one of the simplest and most cost-effective ways to promote health and beauty. Particularly if dry skin is a problem for you, dry brushing is a treat that's not to be missed. Your dry, itchy skin will be gently brushed away, revealing the fresh skin below.

To dry brush, choose a natural bristle brush with soft bristles. You can find an inexpensive one at the health food store, pharmacy, grocery store, or online. They usually have a natural wood handle and come in two different styles. One style fits in the palm of your hand; the other style has a long handle, like a back brush. Body brushes with handles work well on the back of your body, but may be a little difficult to use in close-in areas, such as your feet. For those areas, the palm-sized brush is easier and more comfortable to use. Begin with the softest bristles possible and work your way up to a stiffer bristle. Stiffer bristles, like a cactus-bristle brush, will generate more lymphatic stimulation. If your skin is delicate, you may have to work your way up to a stiffer brush over time, and not use it every day; also be careful around delicate areas.

My friend Theresa has ageless, flawless, wrinkle-free skin, and she's dry brushed her skin, including her face, twice a day for more than 30 years. She has grown children and grandchildren, and her skin rivals any 35-year-old's I know.

Dry brushing style

Dry brushing is basic and easy to do—plus it feels great, like giving yourself a gentle massage. Some tips to make the experience even better:

- Sit or stand on a towel or in your tub or shower stall to collect any dead skin.
- Don't wet your skin or the brush, or you won't get the same benefit.
- Start at the bottom of your feet. It's like a wake-up call to your nerve endings to get ready to be stimulated.
- Brush inward and upward if you can, but this isn't an exact science. You can't do this wrong.
- Move up from the feet to the legs, brushing up toward your torso.
- Start again at your fingertips and move inward toward your heart.
- Be gentle on or avoid your breasts and neck.
- When brushing your stomach and abdominal area, use counter-clockwise strokes to stimulate your digestion.
- I don't recommend brushing your face with a body brush; however, a small, very soft and gentle brush that feels good on your face can work nicely.
- Wash your brush every few weeks and allow it to dry completely before using again.
- You can dry brush up to twice a day, but you'll see benefits even if you brush every other day. If you notice any irritated skin, however, don't brush that area until it returns to normal. Start again with a softer brush.

Other tools for exfoliation include a woven hemp mitt to use with your shower gel, or a loofah mitt. Wet exfoliation doesn't have the same stimulating effect on your lymphatic system as dry brushing.

Your face

Facial skin benefits from exfoliation as well. Brushing or gently scrubbing away dead skin cells as you spring cleanse will give you even more of a glow. Winter can leave your skin pores blocked and dull looking. As your diet improves from your cleanse, so will your skin. You'll want to exfoliate so that your new, healthy skin can enjoy the warmer weather.

Using a natural exfoliation method is a better choice than having polyester fibers treated with chemicals roughing up your gentle epidermis. A natural gentle loofah designed for the face, a small soft skin brush, or an organic cotton washcloth all can gently exfoliate facial skin.

For some added help, you can purchase a natural skin care scrub. You can also mix up your own healthy skin scrub, using my own formulas. The scrub will be absorbed into your skin, so be sure to use only organic, pure ingredients—I get essential oils from doterra.com. Making your own scrub is simple and takes only a few minutes. Your skin will thank you if you try.

Wild Orange Facial Scrub

This scrub is made of cleansing and moisturizing ingredients that support your skin. Raw honey is naturally antibacterial and moisturizing. The finely ground almonds moisturize your skin with their natural oil while helping to gently exfoliate. Sweet almond oil is high in A and B vitamins. It's also naturally moisturizing. The wild orange essential oil is uplifting and cleansing.

Preparation: Combine all the ingredients in a small bowl and mix thoroughly. Smooth a thin layer over your face and then gently rub it off with an organic cotton washcloth, using a circular motion.

Ingredients:

- 3 tbsp local honey
- 3 tbsp finely ground almonds (use a food processor or a coffee grinder that's not used for coffee)
- 3 tbsp sweet almond oil
- 5 drops wild orange essential oil

Flower Garden Honey Scrub with Rose and Geranium

This beautifully scented honey scrub smells like spring; it's a gentle exfoliation that moisturizes and soothes damaged skin. Coconut oil is antibacterial and anti-inflammatory, making this good for inflamed skin. Coconut sugar is a soft and gentle scrub, while honey is moisturizing and antimicrobial. Rose essential oil is particularly beneficial for mature skin and dry, sensitive skin, while geranium essential oil helps soothe inflammation.

Preparation: Combine all the ingredients in a small bowl and mix thoroughly. Smooth a thin layer over your face and then gently rub it off with an organic cotton washcloth, using a circular motion.

Ingredients:

- 3 tbsp coconut oil (gently warmed to liquid)
- 3 tbsp granulated coconut sugar
- 3 tbsp local honey
- 5 drops rose essential oil
- 5 drops geranium essential oil

Ingredients:

1 c Dead Sea salts
1 c baking soda
10 drops lavender essential oil

Lavender Detox Bath

Dead Sea salts are rich in minerals such as calcium, magnesium, potassium, and sulfur. The mixture helps detoxify the body by pulling toxins out and adding in essential minerals. Baking soda softens the skin and neutralizes your body's acidity, while lavender is calming and relaxing to the mind and body. This detox bath is a great way to end your day.

Preparation: Add the ingredients to the water in a hot bath. Swish them around with your hands to mix them into the water.

Essential Oils

All the formulas I just gave you contain essential oils. What are these? They're the natural aromatic compounds found in the seeds, bark, stems, roots, flowers, and other parts of plants. They're made by either steam distilling the plant matter to remove the aromatic substances, or by pressing them, much like squeezing a lemon. The end product is highly concentrated, so you need only a few drops. Despite their name, essential oils aren't oily. They feel clean to the touch.

Because they're water-based and contain volatile organic compounds, essential oils are absorbed into the skin rapidly. To avoid skin irritation, essential oils are usually mixed with a natural oil carrier, such as grape-seed, sesame, or coconut oil. Essential oils are mostly for external use, but many can be taken internally as well. Check with a holistic practitioner to be sure which ones are edible. And although they smell great, they're not perfumes.

Essential oils have been used throughout history in many cultures for their medicinal and therapeutic benefits. Modern scientific study in the twentieth century and current trends toward more holistic approaches have brought more attention to essential oil health applications. It's important to purchase your oils from a reputable company with rigorous standards of purity.

Dozens of essential oils from a wide variety of plants are commonly used therapeutically. A few drops of your favorite added to your bath water makes a long soak even more relaxing. They're also wonderful to add to a massage lotion. In aromatherapy, essential oils are often used for vapor inhalation.

Different essential oils are said to have different effects. Peppermint, for example, is energizing, while lavender is relaxing. Rosemary is said to help enhance the memory.

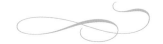

Now that you're revved up, cleaned out, and moving again, let's keep going. Winter is now a distant memory; your skin is glowing and the warm weather beckons you to come out and play. As the rains of spring wind down, you're ready to feel the sun on your shoulders and continue on your healthy path. Summer is calling you to join in the fun. Don't hesitate—there's so much more in store.

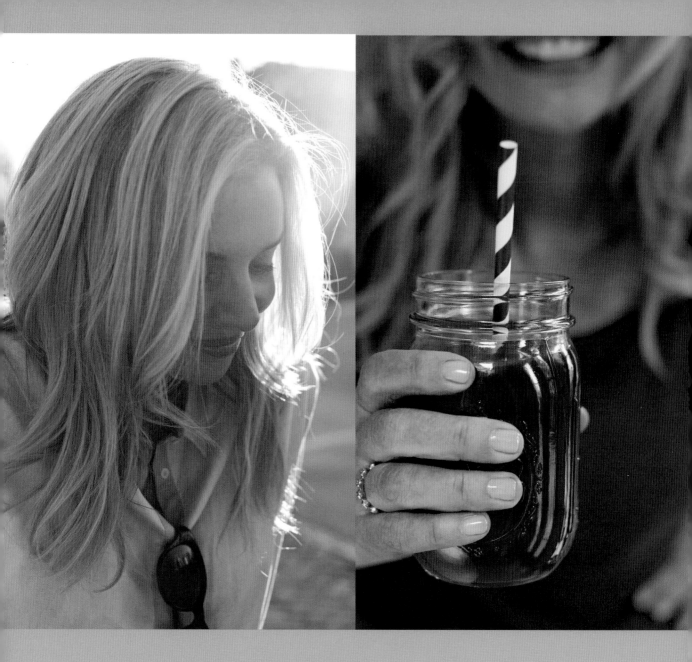

To take advantage of what's near

and local can be the best thing for your overall health, your looks, your energy levels, and your taste buds

Ease into Summer

Feel it coming. Summer eases in with a warm embrace as spring showers subside into full-on sun and the occasional afternoon thunderstorm. You reach for sunglasses and sandals and have a desire to run away from it all, to escape to white sands and ocean breezes. Things slow down as the heat and humidity press in, and no matter what your lifestyle, you need a break from the action. It's time for a vacation—to explore foreign cities, soar across the bay on a sailboat, or hike way up into the mountains and set up camp. Summer calls you to travel somewhere, anywhere, to put your feet up and relax.

If you're more the staycation type, the prospect of quiet days at home feels easier, almost intoxicating. I've given myself several staycations at our farm over the past few years, enjoying a Mediterranean-style life filled with fresh, local foods and long, sunny days in which to enjoy them. My type A personality seems to subside come June, July, and August, as I savor *la dolce vita*. Sometimes I feel downright lazy.

Nothing makes me happier than keeping a gorgeous bowl of summer fruit sitting on my kitchen table, including small green apples from our own apple tree, for my son and his friends. I adore being able to add garden-fresh mint to my iced tea or smoothies, or blend freshly picked tomatoes into a raw sauce for gluten-free or raw zucchini pasta.

I love walking down our country road after dinner or driving out with my husband to see the latest summer movie after a blistering-hot afternoon. My gardener girlfriends begin to reap the rewards of their intense spring planting, showing off raised beds bursting with fresh, colorful produce, and the unwelcome weeds they continuously tackle. (I prefer perennial herbs and the low-maintenance container garden approach.) The back porch with my Mac, two dogs, and three kitties is my favorite place to be. It's my summer office, and I begin each day with a morning tea before the air gets too sultry and the sun too high.

Many businesses, even in the United States, quiet down as executives and assistants alike take their long-awaited time off, or at the very least, dash out the door early on a Friday. Water cooler talk revolves around airfares, beach traffic, and the challenges of sunburn, or whose kid is going to which summer camp. There's a sense of letting go that permeates this time of year and allows you to kick back. Even my high-powered Manhattan executive clients let go this time of year. I highly recommend you embrace the season, too.

Work With the Season, Not Against It

Even though summer seems like a time for the good life, it can have its downside when it comes to how you feel about your looks, your body weight, and finding your own ideal nutrition plan.

Most people's lives bear no resemblance to what we see portrayed in a magazine ad—a perfectly coiffed model dashing off on the Hampton jitney toting a trendy bag. The high heat and humidity can lead to water retention and swelling from an increased salt intake, and belly fat bloat from too many margaritas or diet soft drinks. And since you've sworn off Brazilian straighteners, your hair's frizzy. Swimsuit season can create a disappointing realization of weight gain. Whoops. Summer's the time every year when I come face to face with how much I've been working out . . . or not.

Those go-to foods of summer, like creamy ice cream, seem to be available everywhere, and it can be hard not to cave in and indulge. Your body craves foods to cool down, but having this treat too often can add pounds and cause inflammation from all that sugar and dairy.

The summer heat makes you sweat more. Your body naturally wants salt to help prevent dehydration and replace needed electrolytes. Reaching for tortilla chips and salsa is easy, but some days, within minutes of eating them, you're staring down at puffy hands and fingers.

And when you're on a summer vacation and spending a lot of time outdoors in the heat, it's hard not to give in to cravings. When I was growing up, my family vacationed at the Jersey Shore (yes, I'm a Jersey girl), and I had a daily craving for vanilla soft serve to work its cooling magic. The relief was short-term, however. Inevitably I'd feel sick to my stomach within an hour—it was only years later that I realized this came from my intolerance to dairy and eating too much sugar.

Like birthdays and holidays, summer vacations are the time to have fun and indulge a little.

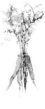

I remember my sister coming in from a day at the beach, grabbing a bag of potato chips, diving in, and saying, "I need salt!" The next morning, she held up her swollen fingers and announced, "Too much salt!"

Like birthdays and holidays, summer vacations are the time to have fun and indulge a little. If you want ice cream from that great little stand on the boardwalk at the beach, go for it. I love to indulge on those special days, although I go for organic sorbet or non-dairy treats instead of ice cream. But what happens on vacation stays on vacation. I've learned that if I behave every day as I do when I'm on vacation, I won't feel and look the way I like. I'll begin to feel lousy, with aches and pains, a foggy brain, and reddish skin.

Get Raw

Summer provides lots of opportunities to give in to your cravings, so let's talk about how to satisfy those natural tendencies without gaining weight and feeling grumpy by September.

Imagine biting into a ripe, fresh plum, or getting a waft of blueberries as you pass by fragrant cartons of them at your farmer's market. Imagine slicing into homegrown strawberries that smell and taste sweet, unlike the mealy out-of-season berries you bought last winter. Smell the peppery, early arugula of June, the intoxicating aroma of July watermelons, or the understated scent of cucumber fresh from your garden in August. Slice into a fresh tomato and remember what a tomato is supposed to smell and taste like. It's easy to forget if you've been eating the grocery store kind all winter.

Summer offers an abundance of delicious fruits and vegetables that can be eaten raw or very lightly cooked. To take advantage of what's near and local can be the best thing for your overall health, your looks, your energy levels, and your taste buds.

What is raw food?

A raw food or a raw food diet refers to foods that are eaten mostly uncooked. If they're cooked, it's very gently—they're not heated to above 115 degrees Fahrenheit. The primary reason for eating raw foods is to preserve intact the natural enzymes in the food. Enzymes are natural proteins made by living cells or animals; enzymes make the normal metabolic processes of the body, such as digestion, happen faster.

Think of raw foods as a complete health kit, with no added ingredients needed for them to do their magic. Plants, like fruits, vegetables, herbs, nuts, and seeds, contain enzymes that, in an uncooked state, will help your body to digest them. Because of this benefit, your body doesn't use its own enzyme reserve to break down and absorb the food, so it doesn't have to work as hard at digestion. If you did the Cleanse with Style protocol outlined in chapter four, you've at least experimented with increasing raw foods in your diet.

Digestive system health is the key to overall health. Seventy percent of your body's power to resist disease rests in your digestive system, making it your first line of defense against bacteria, viruses, and pathogens. Complex processed foods and toxic pesticides and sprays weaken the digestive tract. Because of this, our bodies produce fewer digestive enzymes as we age—enzymes we need to allow us to absorb food's nutrients.

SARAH Fruit Instead of Ice Cream

My client Sarah, a Healthy Omnivore, was addicted to the cold, sweet creaminess of ice cream. Even though she knew she'd feel better if she cut back, Sarah struggled with her craving. She tried switching from high-fat gourmet ice creams with funny names to the popular 100-calorie cones and bars, but she would eat the entire box while driving home from the store. Sarah wasn't terribly overweight; she was more concerned about her health and overall nutrition than the extra 15 pounds she carried. After eating the ice cream, she felt like crap—swollen, puffy, and nauseated. She wanted to break that cycle and ramp up the quality of her nutrition to feel, in her words, "amazing."

We decided Sarah should try swapping fresh fruit for ice cream. I told her, "Take your biggest fruit bowl out of the cupboard, or go buy a huge one, and place it on your kitchen table. Next, visit the farmer's market and buy an assortment of fruits that you love. Smell them, and make sure you really get in touch with their sweetness and freshness. Fill the bowl, and when the craving for ice cream hits, have a piece of fruit. If you still have that craving, have another piece. In fact, eat an unlimited amount of fruit for now, whenever that craving strikes."

Sarah was soon carrying fruit around with her everywhere she went. She had containers of fruit in her car, her handbag, and in a bowl on her desk. Every time that sweet, cold craving hit, she'd eat a piece of fruit.

After just a few days, Sarah began to feel great. Fresh fruit crowded out her ice cream cravings and she quickly dropped a couple of pounds. Her face lost its red, inflamed appearance and her skin had a healthy glow. The joyful thing for me to see was that she was eating seasonal, locally grown fresh fruits and remembering how good real food tasted. And the ice cream? It's not gone forever, but she enjoys it now only as a special occasion dessert.

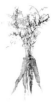

Raw foods are easier to digest because they come with their own enzymes. If your digestion is even slightly compromised, adding in more raw foods can help. Blended smoothies and liquid nutrition are especially helpful, as they save your body the effort of breaking down the food from a solid form. (See the recipes in chapter ten for some great ways to get your liquid nutrition.)

The outward result? People who eat an all-raw diet, or a high percentage of raw foods, often experience a high-level, "go-for-it" kind of energy. They have clear, glowing skin, focused thinking, and an overall sense of well-being. Raw food is anti-aging, pumping in live phytonutrients to your skin cells to provide a vibrant, youthful look.

For some, a raw food diet can be the best way to eat all of the time, or almost all the time. This isn't true for everyone. You won't know how much raw is good for you, however, until you try it. Start gently by adding just a bit more raw food into your daily meals—a salad of fresh greens with both lunch and dinner, some fresh fruit as a snack. In the same way that you tuned in to your body to help discover your Nutritional Style, tune in to how you feel after eating more raw foods. If you're feeling great from the added raw food, gradually move yourself toward a mostly raw or even an all-raw diet.

Summer is the ideal time to experiment with "going raw." We naturally reach for cooling foods in hot weather. In the abundant days of summer, the local markets are bursting with fresh produce. We're instinctively drawn to this array of produce to help us stay cool and also for their cleansing properties. And who wants to cook when it's that hot?

Raw foods are cleansing because they're free of additives or chemicals. A cucumber or tomato or watermelon doesn't come with a label listing the added ingredients. Fruits and vegetables pass through your digestive system with ease, allowing you to assimilate all their nutrients.

Raw vegetables and fruits cool the body naturally. If you're craving sweets, the fruits of summer are here to help. With natural sugars and high-fiber content, fruit sugars are absorbed into your system slowly—you don't get the sugar rush and glycemic spike from sugary snacks such as cookies. Also, you'll find that fruit is much more filling and satisfying. You could probably eat a dozen Oreos at one time, but you most likely can't eat more than two juicy, fresh peaches in a row.

If you're craving the sugar lift and the cooling effect of ice cream, now's the time to reach for some fragrant fresh fruit instead. If you want something cold, try freezing some grapes or orange slices—they make a great snack.

Smoothies are tasty, fast, and economical.

Is Raw Your Nutritional Style?

Some people find eating too many raw vegetables, fruits, nuts, and seeds can be difficult on their digestion, causing gas, bloating, and even diarrhea. If that's the case for you, try blending or juicing your raw foods. This cuts back on the amount of fiber you're adding to your system and lets your digestion adjust to having more raw foods to process. Even if you have a strong digestive system, liquefying large amounts of the plants and their beneficial phytonutrients will be easier on your digestion and allow you to consume more.

Most people who eat large amounts of raw food juice their vegetables and fruits, or blend them into smoothies as part of their daily routine. Green smoothies are a way of getting more greens, and green juice can be a great pick-me-up instead of a caffeinated beverage. You may want to mix it up and enjoy a savory nut-and-veggie pâté blended in your food processor or try some raw dark chocolate desserts, like my 3-minutes-in-the-blender recipe for homemade chocolate truffles. (The recipes are in chapter ten.)

If you're a Modern Vegan, you already incorporate most of these ideas into your diet, and my guess is you love summer for all its raw abundance. Flexible Vegetarians can try to ease back on the heavier cooked legumes and grains and enjoy protein from sprouted seeds and smoothies instead. For Healthy Omnivores, this is a great time to lighten up your diet. Try eating mostly raw foods, including smoothies and salads, until the evening, then enjoy a grilled chicken or fish and vegetable dinner.

I begin each summer day with a smoothie or a juice, deciding each morning whether my body needs the slower absorption of a green smoothie (due to its high fiber content), or the jet-fuel injection of a pressed juice when I want to rev it up. You can discover for yourself when a smoothie or a juice feels best. There's no right way. It's up to your taste buds, your time, and your budget. Smoothies are tasty, fast, and economical. You just toss the whole ingredients into

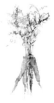

your blender and turn it on. Juicing takes longer to do and uses huge volumes of fruits and vegetables, so it can get expensive fast if you're juicing throughout the day, every day.

Because the natural fiber is mostly removed from fruit juices, the sugar in them hits your system more quickly than eating whole fruit does. If you're sensitive to sugar or have prediabetes or diabetes, fruit juices or green juices with a high fruit content may not be right for you. If you feel an energy crash about an hour after drinking fruit juice, or if you feel bloated or lethargic afterward, skip the juice and go for the whole fruit instead—or go for vegetable smoothies with little or no fruit. One thing to beware of: If you feel an energy crash after a fruit juice or smoothie, that could mean you have blood sugar problems. Check in with your doctor—you may need to head off or treat diabetes.

Sometimes a client of mine will crave sugar in the form of sweets, or starchy carbohydrates, or even fruit. This can be a sign of a yeast infection (candida). If you also have other candida symptoms, such as itchy skin, lethargy, brain fog, or even depression, this could be an issue for you to explore with your doctor.

If you do have blood sugar issues or diabetes, berries, which are plentiful this time of year, are the best choice. In fact, diabetes specialists recommend them. Try to avoid high-sugar tropical fruits, such as pineapple, mango, papaya, and bananas. These fruits are often recommended as additions to sweeten vegetable juices. If you can't handle them, though, switch up your veggie blend instead. Cut back on the dark leafy greens such as kale and add more romaine, cucumber, or celery; adding lemon juice, ginger, and stevia will help to sweeten the blend.

Raw Food Week

If you want to give eating raw a try, you might want to experiment with an all-raw day and use some raw recipes from this book, or eat raw foods most of the day and enjoy a cooked dinner. I often do this, sipping a green juice or creamy smoothie for breakfast, eating a crisp green salad loaded with superfoods (hemp seeds, seaweed, pumpkin seeds, etc.) for lunch, and later enjoying a lightly sautéed dinner of fresh veggies from the garden with quinoa.

If you're feeling ready for it, go for a raw food week. As well as being a fun experiment in a different way of eating, a raw food week is also a great way to cleanse after a vacation splurge.

Preparing raw food takes some extra time. Get ready for your raw food clean-eating week by shopping, blending, and preparing ahead of time. Not too far ahead, because you want your fruits and veggies to be nice and fresh. Eating raw does take a bit of extra work, too—some recipes can be complex and time-consuming to prepare. If you're really pressed for time, check out the raw food delivery services I list in the resources section at the back of this book.

Protein

A raw food diet is close to what we're calling a Modern Vegan diet in this book—leaving out most animal products (with the exception of honey), and eliminating cooked beans, legumes, and most grains, with the exception of those that are raw and sprouted. Without the standard plant sources of protein, can you get enough of this crucial nutrient on a raw food diet?

Protein sources for a raw diet include nuts, seeds, and dark leafy greens. Most raw foodists add in copious amounts of greens (kale, chard, spinach, etc.) to provide plenty of protein, vitamins, and minerals. They blenderize their foods to allow their bodies to digest those amounts needed for ultimate health. Raw foodists and most Modern Vegans are keenly aware of the nutritional values of their foods and keep an arsenal of superfoods on hand to ensure their success.

By using raw food preparation methods such as blending and juicing, and through their directed focus on nutrition, people who eat a lot of raw food usually get plenty of easily assimilated protein. Following a raw food diet strengthened my nails and my hair. My nails started to grow in again, after years of breakage. In an ah-ha moment at a hair salon in New York, I realized that after a year of eating raw, my hair was long and thick again.

Some people actually go so far as to include raw fish and meat in their raw foods eating plan, but that's not something I'm comfortable recommending. Sushi is fine when it's prepared from really fresh fish at a good restaurant by skilled chefs, but otherwise, avoid raw animal foods—the inevitable bacteria on them could make you really sick.

Following a raw food diet strengthened my nails and my hair.

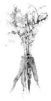

Adding in raw foods to your menu will also allow you to push out other foods, such as processed cereals, breads, and animal protein. All of these foods can slow and clog your digestion and lower your energy levels. The more efficient your digestion is, the more efficiently your body works. Use summer as an easy, delicious pass to a healthy way of eating.

Crowd out the junk; ditch the processed foods for breakfast and enjoy a big bowl of berries, or a green smoothie with fresh fruit included. Forget the sandwich for lunch and instead grab a fresh salad topped with easy-to-digest avocado slices and hemp seeds. Try raw zucchini pasta a few nights a week and discover if eating the raw way adds some spring to your step.

Discovering your Nutritional Style is about finding what works for you. Maybe raw is your summer Nutritional Style?

Hydration

You don't need me to tell you to drink more water; your body lets you know right away when you need it, right? Wrong! Your body doesn't signal to you that you're thirsty until you're already a bit dehydrated, and by then your cells already have started to wilt. Symptoms of mild dehydration include foggy brain and low energy—maladies that most people try to fix with caffeine (a diuretic that makes dehydration worse).

Besides giving you more vroom-vroom and clearer thinking, being properly hydrated helps sustain a youthful appearance. Water plumps your cells and adds elasticity, resulting in softer, smoother, younger-looking and glowing skin. That's a train I want to be riding on!

Properly hydrated internal cells help keep your body functioning at its best. Just as eating raw foods aids digestion, so does drinking plenty of water. You want to stay hydrated so that you can take full advantage of the nutrients in the organic foods you so mindfully found and prepared.

Drinking more water also helps with weight loss. It works in three primary ways: water helps keep your digestion efficient, reduces hunger, and curbs cravings.

The summer season is packed with fresh vegetables and fruits that all seem to be superfoods. They are, but some are more super than others. In the summer, if you have to choose, pick these:

Carrots

Most carrots are orange, but did you know that heirloom varieties also come in purple, yellow, red, and white? Each color offers a different variety of powerful antioxidants, a great reason to explore local farmers' markets when they're in season. Known for their high beta carotene content, carrots help prevent oxidative damage and are beneficial in preventing cardiac disease, too. High in vitamin A, biotin, and vitamin K, and loaded with fiber, they're gorgeous powerhouses of nutrition. Be sure to pull the fresh greens off the tops prior to storing them, as the greens will pull the moisture from the carrot root, causing them to wilt. (This goes for radishes, too.) We love them steamed lightly and served with herbs and a touch of local honey. We also love our Bunny Juice, a carrot blend that I make a few times a week.

Broccoli

Doesn't everyone love this veggie? It's a delicious stand-by with superpower nutritional benefits. A cup of broccoli has more than a full day's requirements of vitamins C and K, and is a good source of vitamin A, chromium, and folate. Broccoli should be lightly steamed to retain its strong nutrient profile; steaming also enhances its cholesterol-lowering benefits. I add broccoli florets to gluten-free pasta to please a posse of boys, and create an easy blended soup from steamed broccoli, broth, onions, and herbs.

Tomatoes

These are my dad's favorite, and he swears that his Jersey tomatoes are the best. Far be it from me to argue with him. A staple in Italian cuisine, tomatoes are off the charts in the phytonutrient department, offering high levels of beta carotene, lycopene, and numerous heart-health benefits. They're high in vitamins A, C, and K, and biotin. To keep their texture, tomatoes should be stored at room temperature (just ask my Dad), but once ripe, refrigerating them for a day or two will help keep them fresh. Like peppers and eggplants, tomatoes are in the nightshade family. Some people feel foods from this family cause inflammation and joint pain. If you have joint issues, you might wish to remove nightshades for two weeks to see how you feel. It's possible you're sensitive to them.

Cucumber

Cucumbers are a personal favorite; light and unassuming, they overrun the garden in late July and August. They're high in antioxidants, helping to reduce free radicals, and they're anti-inflammatory as well. Cucumber skin contains silica, a moisturizing benefit that helps with joint issues and hydrates your skin. Cucumbers also provide electrolytes that are much needed in the hot summer months when they grow (Mother Nature is so savvy). They also contain vitamin C, beta carotene, and manganese. Puree cucumbers, tomatoes, peppers, and a few spring onions for a quick gazpacho, or do what I do: Add them to your juice or green smoothie daily. Just be sure to use organic produce and leave the skins on.

Blueberries

When I learned that blueberries improve memory, I wanted to add them to my diet every day. They also help to regulate blood sugar and are high in a variety of phytonutrients, as well as vitamin D, vitamin K, manganese, and fiber. Try to eat your blueberries fresh and raw to maintain their juicy nutrients. Freezing them works well, too, especially in the summer when they're abundant and you have extra. Fresh or frozen blueberries make great smoothies, by themselves or with other fruits.

Water aids digestion (and therefore your metabolism) by helping your body produce sufficient stomach acids to digest and assimilate nutrients. Efficient digestion may mean you don't have as many cravings for unhealthy foods. Sufficient water allows the body to move waste by keeping everything soft and easy to pass; it also helps keep the linings of the stomach and intestinal walls healthy.

Drinking water prior to meals or snacks reduces hunger by creating a feeling of fullness. Staying hydrated also prevents water retention and bloating. When the body is short on water, it retains what it has. Even though it may seem counterintuitive, summer bloat and puffy hands are actually a call to drink more water. When properly hydrated, your body's metabolism remains regulated and, *voila!*, you're wearing your favorite shoes and cocktail rings, and you may never have to feel puffy again.

Being hydrated also helps to curb cravings. Often when we think we're hungry, we're actually thirsty, so drinking water before meals and in-between, before cravings set in, could mean that you skip that bag of pretzels or chips.

It might seem far-reaching to give so much credit to something so simple, but if you're not drinking at least 64 ounces of water a day, especially in the summer heat, you're most likely facing some of the symptoms I've mentioned. The amount of water recommended for daily consumption varies, but experts generally agree that it depends on your body weight, your activity level, and the time of year. Adding in some extra water is very easy to do, so it's worth a try. Once again, tune in to what works for you. One clear way to see if you're properly hydrated, other than checking in on your energy, hunger, and whether or not your rings fit, is to check your urine. If you're drinking enough, your urine will be a very pale yellow. If it's yellow or dark yellow, you're suffering from a lack of water. Drink up!

Special factors like illness, pregnancy, breast-feeding, extreme sports, or long periods outdoors in high heat all call for additional hydration. If that's you, 64 ounces a day, or the 8 x 8 formula (8 ounces of water 8 times a day) is an easy one to remember. It's a good starting guideline for discovering your personal hydration style.

For me, staying hydrated has to be a conscious effort each day. Like you, I'm busy. I can easily forget to stop what I'm doing and have a glass of water or iced herbal tea. On the days when I don't bother to drink enough for good hydration, I can see and feel the difference. I get tired and cranky. I have to make a conscious decision to step back and ask myself why I feel that way. Too often, it's because the water pitcher on my desk is still half-full. When you find yourself feeling irritable or wondering if you can squeeze in a quick nap, ask yourself if you've had enough to drink so far. You might be surprised at how quickly a cup of herbal tea or a glass of water improves your mood and perks up your energy level.

Balancing Electrolytes

Electrolytes are the necessary minerals that control the fluid balance of your body. The amount of sodium (salt), potassium, chloride, calcium, magnesium, and bicarbonate in your blood and in the fluid between your cells is crucial for maintaining the basic metabolic processes in your body. Because an electrolyte imbalance can be very dangerous, your body constantly monitors your levels. Your kidneys, for instance, keep the electrolyte concentrations in your blood constant by reabsorbing minerals from your urine and reducing or increasing the amount of urine you make. Your electrolytes can get out of balance and put a lot of extra stress on your body if your fluid and mineral outgo isn't balanced by intake. When you play a long tennis match on a hot day, for instance, you sweat, which means you lose water and minerals. You might get dehydrated enough to have muscle cramps or feel woozy. If you're outdoors a lot in hot weather or if you're physically active enough to sweat a lot at any time of year, carry that water bottle with you—and drink it.

ANNA Hydration for Weight Loss

My client Anna had trouble losing weight and she was retaining water like crazy. Anna was sure it was hereditary, because her mother also had complained of swelling. When I asked Anna how much water she drank each day, I was surprised at how low the amount was. Anna thought that her green smoothie, all 32 ounces of it, would do the trick for her daily hydration needs.

I gave her some easy ways to add more water throughout the day. Anna began by drinking a quart-sized pitcher of water flavored with lemon and stevia each morning and another one after lunch. She learned to enjoy herbal teas and added them to her day, instead of coffee and tea. Anna quickly shed the puffiness—and her energy increased as well. It made a profound difference to her weight and her overall outlook on life. She shared that tip with her mom and bought her a pretty glass water pitcher to go along with it.

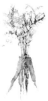

Commercial energy drinks, sports drinks, and vitamin water are marketed as a great source of electrolytes. I don't recommend them. They do have added minerals, but they also contain large amounts of sugar in the form of high-fructose corn syrup, mixed in with unhealthy additives and artificial coloring. You can replenish more naturally and less expensively simply by drinking water and eating a piece of fruit or having a small amount of fruit juice. Fruit is a great natural source of potassium, the most important mineral to replace when you're dehydrated. Citrus fruits contain natural electrolytes, so cutting up oranges for your daughter's big game makes sense. (For a homemade electrolyte drink that's easy to make, see the summer recipes in chapter ten.)

Coconut water is another great option. Just a third of a cup of fresh coconut water has 250 mg of potassium and 105 mg of sodium, enough to replenish what you've lost in a heavy workout. Fill the rest of the glass with pure water to replace the water you've sweated out.

Simple ways to get more water into your day

I'm guilty of skimping on the water even when my pitcher is sitting reproachfully right in front of me, so I've become something of an expert on finding ways to get more water into my day. Some ideas that have worked for me and my clients:

Treat yourself to some new water bottles and fill them up each morning as you prepare your breakfast. (You can do this the night before, too.) Put one in your tote, one in your car, and one on your desk. Be sure your bottle is glass (my preference for you), stainless steel, or BPA-free plastic.

If you work at home, fill a lovely 32-ounce pitcher and put it somewhere conspicuous on your work area. If you see it, you'll drink it. In hot summer weather, aim to drink two pitchers a day. At least.

Don't get in the car, subway, metro, bus, train, or on a plane without carrying at least one full bottle of water.

Take a large bottle of water with you to your workout. Drink a third of it on the way to the gym, another third when you take a breather, and finish it off when after you end the workout.

Drink a glass of water prior to a meal. This has a double advantage: It hydrates you while cutting your appetite.

FLAVOR UP YOUR WATER

Tired of boring, plain water? Try adding one of these combinations to a pitcher of filtered water and savor it all day.

- Cardamom, star anise, and cinnamon sticks for a spicy winter drink
- Pomegranate seeds and a small amount of fresh pomegranate juice
- Lime slices, mint, and maple syrup for a "virgin mojito"
- Cucumber slices for a gentle hint of flavor
- Edible lavender blossoms and three drops of liquid lemon stevia
- Orange or clementine slices, gently squeezed, with strawberry slices
- Frozen raspberries, blackberries, or blueberries for a powerful burst of antioxidant flavor
- Fresh, crushed mint leaves and a splash of fresh nectarine or clementine juice
- Three drops flavored liquid stevia, such as chocolate or vanilla cream, and a dash of cinnamon
- Swedish bitters aid digestion and are a great mocktail when added to sparkling water
- Peppermint essential oil and a drop of liquid stevia for "candy cane" water
- Cayenne pepper and lemon slices for hot and spicy lemonade to boost the metabolism
- Cinnamon and lemon slices for sweet and spicy lemonade
- Maple syrup, lime, and cayenne pepper for a cleansing day
- Ripe mango slices and a drop of liquid stevia
- Star fruit slices to decorate water and add delicate flavor
- Celery stick and a slice of lemon for refreshment
- Frozen pineapple chunks; mash one chunk for added juice
- Puréed berries frozen in ice cube trays
- Dash of vanilla and a cinnamon stick for an exotic drink
- Shredded ginger and lemon slices
- A peppermint tea bag or any herbal tea of your choice
- Grapefruit essential oil for weight loss
- Apple cider vinegar and honey for ultimate health
- Dried goji berries for a superfood treat

Flavor it up. Frankly, as much as I know plain water is the best and cheapest way to hydrate, it gets boring. Make something tasty that you'll want to drink. See the list above for ways to spice up your water!

Invest in a mini soft-cooler bag to store your drinks for on the go, especially for hot days. Here's a good tip for when you're going to be outdoors in the heat: The night before, fill a water bottle about a quarter of the way with water and put it in the freezer. When you're ready to go, add more water, leaving some room at the top. Your water will stay nice and cold.

Quality is everything

In the same way that you pay attention to buying organic foods and local, seasonal fare, choose your water wisely.

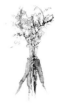

Your kitchen tap might be your best, cheapest source of water, although I recommend filtering your drinking water at the very least. The American municipal water supply is relatively safe in terms of bacteria and creepy-crawlies—waterborne illnesses are very rare here. What's more concerning is the possible presence of other contaminants, such as lead, pesticides, and industrial chemicals. You may be able to find out what's in your municipal water by asking whoever provides your water. The problem might not be there, however—your tap water can pick up contaminants on its way to you or from your plumbing. To be on the safe side, you can have your water tested, usually for free, by your local health department.

Or you can just filter your water. The simplest and least expensive filters use activated carbon. They fit into water pitchers or on the tap or can be installed under the sink. You can also look into

ROSE   Moving Toward Health

My client Rose is a busy dentist with two young children. Her Nutritional Style needed tweaking, but it wasn't horrible at all. As a dentist, she was well aware of the dangers of sugar! Rose was convinced that something was missing from her diet; she was looking for a magic superfood that would change everything and give her back her sparkle.

I worked with Rose over a few months. We ramped up her nutrition, but the key for Rose, the real magic super ingredient, came when she began to move her body.

Rose had been working with a trainer two days a week. She was sure that this was all she could squeeze in to her busy life. I had a hunch that Rose needed more movement and a physical release from the tight confines of her dental office. When we pulled her day apart to search for windows of exercise opportunity, we discovered she had some extra time most mornings after walking her children to summer camp. I asked her, "What if you kept walking for half an hour longer? Could you still make it to the office on time?"

"Sure," she answered, before making excuses: Is

it worth it? will that be enough to make a difference? what if it's raining? and so on. We agreed that she would at least give it a try for a few days.

Rose started the next day, and when we spoke again two weeks later, she said she felt like a new woman. She had found the perfect walking place near her home. She brought her dog along, and the two would head out, with her water bottle, for at least a half hour.

By the time we finished working together, Rose had progressed to running for half an hour. Her new morning habit improved her outlook, gave her quality time for herself, and made her feel bright and happy. We both were thrilled—and so was the dog.

At the end of our final session, after reviewing her new eating plan and recapping her strategy going forward, I remembered that she hadn't shared with me whether her weight had changed. She'd lost 15 pounds! I laughed; her goal in coming to me had been to lose weight, but she felt so good about everything else that her weight loss became the healthy byproduct of her new active lifestyle.

reverse osmosis filters that fit under the sink and remove more contaminants than charcoal filters do. Whole-house filtration systems are installed where your main water pipe enters the house.

Distilling water is an option I like, although it's controversial because it removes all minerals from the water. If you have a good diet full of fruits and veggies, the amount this removes doesn't really matter.

Test your drinking water regularly for toxins, metals, and contaminants to assess your household needs, and get the best water filter you can afford. Then be sure to change the filter regularly, to avoid reintroducing contaminants.

After you've taken the time to test and filter your water, don't forget to use it. At home, use filtered water to make tea and coffee, and for cooking. Send your child to school or camp with a fun water bottle filled with water you're confident is clean and pure, and take your own with you. Don't leave home without it.

Don't fall for advertising about bottled water from some exotic place. It's not healthier—in fact, there's a good chance it's plain tap water in a fancy bottle. Ounce for ounce, bottled water costs more than gasoline. Literally billions of plastic water bottles are discarded each year, resulting in an environmental disaster that future generations will have to clean up. Plastic bottles contain toxins that can leach into the water; when you drink from a plastic water bottle, you're drinking those toxins down.

Summer Movement Style

With more vacation time, and possibly shorter workdays, the summer is the perfect time to move more, while soaking up sunlight to help you make lots of vitamin D. Most of my clients find it easier to get out and be active in summer, mainly because everyone feels better with more sunlight. The luxury of longer days for walking outside in the evenings or enjoying an early-morning run before work is a short-lived gift. If the idea of exercise challenges you, but you have a strong desire to be healthy, vibrant, younger-looking, and toned, the summer is a great time to begin.

Summer Beauty Style

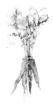

Your long-term beauty style depends in large part on exposure to the sun. In summer, when the sun is at its fiercest, it's crucial to protect your skin safely and consistently.

Most Americans are now aware of the sun's harmful effects: wrinkles, spots, sunburn, and skin cancer. When it comes to your looks, there's no denying that the sun speeds aging and that avoiding facial exposure will keep it looking younger longer. No amount of moisturizer will undo the damage from that weekend sunburn, so take care to cover up with a wholesome, safe sunscreen, and a hat if you're at the beach or in direct sun for extended periods.

Most people are aware of the need for sun protection, yet the most deadly skin cancer, melanoma, is on the rise, with diagnosed cases increasing each year. The reason for this is unclear, but some health advocates believe that it's due to certain toxic ingredients found in the most widely used sunscreens. More likely, it's because people don't use enough sunscreen, don't apply it often enough, or choose a sunscreen that blocks only UVB radiation, and not also the more dangerous UVA radiation.

The Environmental Working Group (EWG), my favorite go-to source for information about this sort of stuff, offers a sunscreen guide that gauges sunscreen effectiveness and evaluates the safety of ingredients. One controversial ingredient, oxybenzone, has a high risk of causing cellular and biochemical changes, according to the EWG. The EWG website (ewg.org) lists the safest, most effective sunscreens and also has a tool for looking up sunscreens and seeing how they rate.

People who supplement sunscreen protection with clothing or hats seem to get fewer sunburns than those who rely solely on sun block. The research shows that avoiding sunburn and tanning beds plays a role in reducing your risk of skin cancer. Studies also have shown that adequate vitamin D levels help to prevent skin cancer, so a limited amount of sun exposure to stimulate your natural production of vitamin D is recommended for optimal health.

The bottom line for your summer sun beauty? Get some sun, but limit your exposure. Use a safe sunscreen (see the resources section at the back of this book for a guide), apply it often, and cover up, too.

Vitamin D

Summer sun can boost your immune system and mood, as well as help you prevent deadly diseases, if you approach it safely. Sunshine boosts your body's production of vitamin D.

Most doctors are now testing their patients for low vitamin D levels for good reason. The sunshine vitamin, as vitamin D is sometimes called, is actually produced in your body through a complex process that begins with natural sunlight on your skin. Get plenty of sunshine and you make plenty of vitamin D. Unfortunately, most of us don't get enough sun. In the colder weather, the sun isn't very strong, the days are short, and we're mostly indoors out of the cold. Even in warmer weather, we spend a lot of time during the day indoors. We're at work, at school, commuting, or staying inside in the air conditioning. Combine that with fear of skin cancer and heavy use of sun blockers, and it's easy to see how a lot of us end up on the low side for vitamin D.

That's a problem, because low vitamin D levels are associated with many health problems. You need plenty of vitamin D to maintain strong bones, keep your immune system strong, reduce your risk of cancer (especially colon cancer and breast cancer), keep your blood pressure down, and help prevent heart disease. Vitamin D can boost your serotonin, one of the feel-good chemicals your brain produces, so it may help relieve depression and anxiety.

Ask your doctor to check your vitamin D levels with a simple blood test called the 25-hydroxy test. A surprising number of people, even those who are outdoors a fair amount, are on the low side. Optimally, you want your level to be between 50 and 70 nanograms per milliliter (ng/ml). It is possible to have too much vitamin D, so you don't want your level to go over 100 ng/ml. People who are indoors a lot, who live in northern regions without a lot of sunshine, and who are overweight are at greater risk for being deficient.

The best way to boost your vitamin D level is to get sunshine on your skin for about twenty minutes a day, preferably between 10:00 a.m. and 2:00 p.m., when the sun is brightest. That's not always possible, of course—and I don't recommend tanning beds. Few foods have a lot of natural vitamin D in them. It's mostly found in egg yolks and oily fish, such as salmon, mackerel, tuna, and sardines. There's also some in cheese, but most people get their vitamin D

> Vitamin D can boost your serotonin, one of the feel-good chemicals your brain produces, so it may help relieve depression and anxiety.

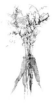

from milk, which by law has vitamin D added to it. It's also added to some breakfast cereals and orange juice, but that cereal is processed and the orange juice isn't really fresh. The milk is most likely not organic, so these are not the healthiest ways to solve this problem.

If you don't eat these foods—and even if you do—consider taking vitamin D supplements in the form of vitamin D3, also called cholecalciferol. This is the form your body absorbs best.

Your body can store vitamin D, but even if you get a lot of summer sun, it's probably not enough to carry you through into the winter. A supplement is a good idea for backup. In the warm weather, I walk out of my office each day at lunchtime to turn my head to the sun. It's relaxing, centering, and calming.

The Sun, for Better or Worse

Summer is a time for enjoying yourself in the sun. Enjoyable and healthy as that is, the sun is also damaging to your skin and hair. You don't have to live indoors in the summer. Instead, try these special DIY formulas to repair sun damage the natural way.

My Favorite Hair Mask

Ingredients:

1/2 c coconut oil
1/2 c olive oil
6 drops lavender essential
oil (optional)

Years ago, when I had a hard time finding clean, organic hair products that work, I stopped relying on store-bought deep-conditioning products for my hair. Today, choices abound, but I often turn to my standby homemade hair mask because it's so easy and I always have it on hand. This mask is perfect for summer hair. It penetrates and softens dry, parched, bleached-out strands.

I comb this through my hair prior to shampooing, and leave it on for as long as I can, sometimes for hours, other times for just 10 minutes. It's so easy!

Preparation: Mix the oils together in a bowl; the olive oil will help to break down the coconut oil and make it easier to spread. Add lavender oil if you like. Comb through your hair, leave on for at least 10 minutes, and rinse off.

Ingredients:

1 c pure aloe vera gel
40 drops lavender essential oil
20 drops Roman chamomile essential oil

After-Sun Savior

When I was 13 years old and visiting my best friend in Florida, I got a terrible sunburn. My friend's wise mother went outside, cut a leaf from the aloe plant, sliced it open, and instructed me and my sunburned friends to apply the sap inside to our skin often. I watched in awe as the aloe healed my tender, blistered skin. When I arrived back home, I swore to never burn again. I was in my early teens when I began using sunscreen and aloe, and I'm happy to say that I'm still a huge fan.

This mix is wonderful for soothing sunburns. Lavender and Roman chamomile are both soothing and anti-inflammatory to the body. If you want a spray instead of a gel, use aloe vera juice and keep it refrigerated in a glass spray bottle. Aloe vera gel and juice are found in health food stores. Try to find an organic brand. It's always best to store aloe in a glass container, rather than plastic—chemicals from the plastic can leach into your juice.

Preparation: Mix gently and store in the refrigerator, covered. Spread a thin layer over sunburned skin.

Ingredients:

1 c castile liquid soap
2 tbsp grape seed oil
20 drops of any essential oil

Summer Shower Wash

This shower soap is so easy and fun to create; you can vary the essential oils according to your mood. I use Dr. Bronner's Pure-Castile Soap (found in any health food store) as a base. Sometimes I crave the bright and sunny citrus smell of lemons, especially in summer, and other times the soothing notes of lavender. My guys love peppermint to wake them up.

Preparation: Combine all the ingredients in a pump bottle. Shake gently to mix. You can store this in the shower, and use just as you would any store-bought shower wash.

Organic Bug Spray

One of the reasons that I'm not a big gardener is that I'm a magnet for biting bugs, whatever kind happens to be around. Just yesterday I was sitting on the back steps, and within 20 minutes I was covered with red welts and itchy bites. My husband, who had been outside pruning all morning long, stared and shook his head in wonder.

I've read that being attractive to biting bugs might have to do with a higher body temperature (I run cold), pregnancy (not right now), alcohol use (unless someone spiked my morning tea, no again), or having type O blood. Bingo! We have a winner.

No matter what the reason, for me gardening, weeding, pruning, or just going for a summer walk result in red welts and itchy bites all over. That is, unless I remember my very own do-it-yourself bug spray.

I've found that you need to refresh this on your skin more often than commercial brands of bug spray, but it does a great job of repelling biting insects.

Preparation: Combine the water, witch hazel, or vinegar, and the essential oil(s) in a spray bottle. Shake well to mix. Spray generously over all exposed skin (except your face).

Ingredients:

1 c water

1 c witch hazel or apple cider vinegar

50 drops essential oil of your choice, or a combination

Summer Kitchen Bug Spray

Country living often comes with ants, and our home is no exception, especially in the summer. I resist having anyone spray toxic insecticides—in addition to the people in the house, we also have a house full of dogs and kitties, and toxic chemicals aren't good for anyone. We also care deeply about keeping an organic household. I discovered these nontoxic ant remedies, and they really work to repel the little critters.

My sister lives in Florida, and like me, she and her husband, Joe, are concerned about toxins in their environment—but they also have an ant problem. Lea sprinkles cinnamon powder around the entrances to her home, and then pushes the cinnamon into the cracks so it's not visible. No ants! The bonus is that on rainy days, their home smells faintly of cinnamon. It's divine!

Preparation: Combine all the ingredients in a spray bottle and shake well to mix. Lavender, peppermint, and cinnamon all repel ants. Spray wherever you see ants.

Ingredients:

1 tsp liquid dish soap

1 tsp olive oil or grape seed oil

4 c water

40 drops lavender, peppermint, or cinnamon essential oil, alone or in combination

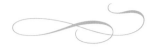

Summer can be a beautiful gift for your health, if you take advantage of everything it has to offer. (For that matter, if you live in a warm climate year-round you may want to memorize this seasonal chapter!) So this is your reminder to shop your seasonal produce markets, get out into the sunshine with a safe sunscreen and move, and enjoy all the gifts that nature gives us right now, before the weather turns chilly and life gets in the way. It's the time to boost your nutrition with more raw foods and fresh ingredients, and maybe even explore a new Nutritional Style.

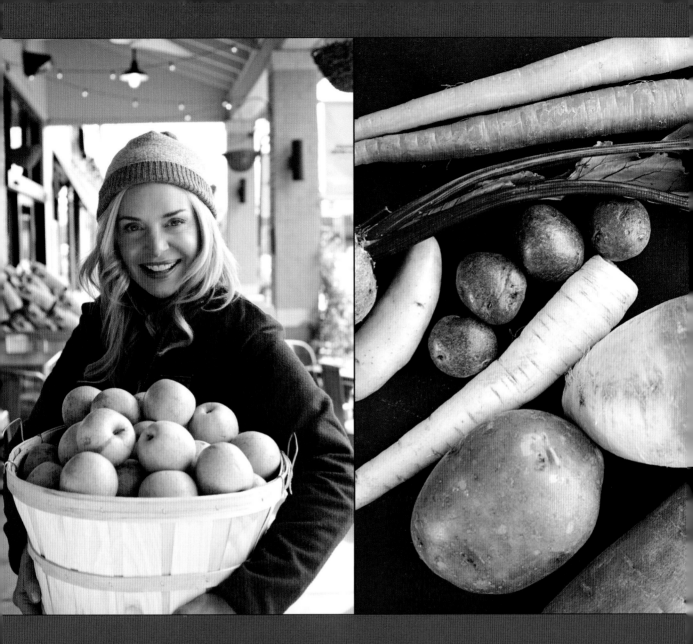

Your Nutritional Style can change
not just from year to year but from season to season,
so the start of fall is a great time
to reevaluate your needs.

CHAPTER EIGHT

Autumn Arrives

The clear autumn air crackles with energy, and the sun slants low in the sky. Gorgeous amber hues cast a golden light that signals the arrival of fall, with winter not far behind. Red, orange, and vibrant yellow foliage is breathtaking, and every color seems reflected back in chrysanthemums, pumpkins, and squash of every size and shade.

You're on the move now, managing to-do lists and an overbooked calendar bulging with both work and personal demands. Labor Day is a distant memory; your white clothes are now deep in the back of the closet. These days, you grab a tweed blazer and zoom out the door.

Vacations are over for now. School buses clog the streets, and traffic slows to a commuter crawl as people return to work. At the office, it's time to produce results and bring the year to a successful close. As if that weren't enough, the holidays loom.

Halloween decorations and loose bags of candy tempt you from the checkout lines at the grocery store, quickly changing over to Christmas trees, candy canes, and colored lights. Mom and Dad want to know if they're invited for Thanksgiving, and if your aunt and uncle can come too. You've got travel to arrange and parent-teacher meetings to attend. The thought of needing to buy holiday gifts, even though it's only October, has you reaching for a glass of wine.

Reality hits abruptly when you realize that the expensive summer vacation didn't strengthen you, it exhausted you. Perhaps you veered too far off your Nutritional Style, and maybe your fitness program, too; you're not feeling up to the monumental tasks at hand. You worry that your energy isn't where it needs to be, and your focus weakens as your stress levels rise. You need to be on your A game, and you want to have fun, too, but it all seems impossible. Let's talk about how you can get into your autumn groove and restore your verve.

The Fall Cleanse

Like spring, fall is a good time of year to cleanse. Fall cleansing helps us prepare for the winter months by strengthening and building immunity. Cleansing helps eliminate toxins that can weaken and compromise the immune system, and with the holidays looming, we want to get ready fast. It's a good way to get rid of any accumulated toxins from summer vacation excesses—the cleanse can help you get back on track.

A fall cleanse can help clear the mind and sharpen focus, enabling you to tackle everything on your plate right now. Cleansing also may help shed a few pounds before the holiday season starts, and allow you to not only look fantastic, but feel it, too, for holiday parties.

If you notice little signs of imbalance as life switches into high gear, slow down and check for the early warning signs again—tired, achy joints, seasonal allergies, headaches, exhaustion, and depression can all be signs that your nutrition patterns have faltered and it's time to bring healthy eating back. A nutritional cleanse will give your body a break and help fortify and prepare it for this busy season.

Start by evaluating how many inflammatory foods are currently in your diet. Admit it, at least some sugar, gluten, dairy, alcohol, processed foods, soy, and coffee have crept back into your diet. Are you having any of these foods daily? Weekly? If you did the Nutritional Style cleanse in the spring and were able to give up these foods for two weeks, how do you feel right now compared to when you came off your cleanse?

If you notice a marked difference, and if these foods have gradually returned to your daily fare, then a fall cleanse would be a wise idea.

You'll want to follow the same protocol I outlined in chapter four. Remember the easy substitutions you used to deal with cravings, like blending your own chocolate truffles instead of snatching that grocery store candy bar, or adding quinoa pilaf to your menu so you can skip the bread.

Remember back to how young and fresh your face looked after giving up alcohol for two weeks, and how much softer your skin seemed when you added water and cut back on your coffee. I'd bet you'd love to have that clear, glowing skin back in time for December, when the holiday parties begin.

If you haven't done a cleanse before, autumn is a good time. Time your cleanse so you'll be done before the holiday crunch hits—and so you'll look your best in time for all those parties.

Your Nutritional Style can change not just from year to year, but from season to season, so the start of fall is a great time to reevaluate your needs. If your spring cleanse was geared toward one Nutritional Style, now might be the appropriate time to explore a different style of cleanse. If you're doing a cleanse for the first time, go with your basic Nutritional Style, but be prepared to find that when it's over, your style has changed. If you're a Healthy Omnivore and have added in more plant-based meals since spring, this may be the perfect time to do the Flexible Vegetarian cleanse, continuing to emphasize more beans, lentils, and gluten-free whole grains. The Flexible Vegetarian cleanser will enjoy more liquid nutrition meals daily, while consuming less animal protein than the Healthy Omnivore plan.

Perhaps as a Flexible Vegetarian you've added more raw food and juicing to your diet; this style of eating suits you for now, and you're feeling light and energized. Try the Modern Vegan cleanse this time around for even deeper cleansing. Make two liquid meals a day, and eat a mostly raw food diet, free of animal protein altogether.

Warm It Up

In the same way that the high heat of summer made you crave cooling foods, the chillier weather in fall signals that you need warming foods. As your body adjusts to lower temperatures, you may be drawn to foods that create a warming effect from the inside out. Cold drinks and frozen treats, even healthy ones, may lose their appeal in favor of hot teas and steaming cocoa.

The cleansing, light vegetables of spring, such as tender asparagus and artichokes, and the cooling produce of summer, such as watermelon, berries, and crisp summer squash, are a distant memory. The fall harvest is at its peak and markets are bulging with seasonal, local produce and an abundance of fruits and vegetables in an array of rich orange and red hues.

In the same way you emphasized light vegetables for your spring cleanse, cleansing foods for fall center on heartier, more substantial vegetables. Fall veggies offer stick-to-your-ribs satisfaction and

> As your body adjusts to lower temperatures, you may be drawn to foods that create a warming effect from the inside out.

warmth, fortifying and preparing your body for the colder months. Once again, Mother Nature knows what she's doing.

Autumn squashes, such as butternut, acorn, or spaghetti, or seasonal pumpkin, flavored naturally with spices, are an easy way to curb cravings for carbohydrates this time of year. They provide warming satisfaction. These high-fiber, naturally sweet veggies can be a delicious meal that will help you cleanse and live happily with your Nutritional Style intact.

Root vegetables are plentiful, too. Carrots, onions, turnips, parsnips, and beets are all sweet vegetables that add flavor to your cooking and help to ground your energy right now.

Cleansing Foods for Fall

For your fall cleanse, eat local and seasonal vegetables and fruits wherever possible. Enjoy an abundance of warm foods. If you're preparing a raw food recipe, such as soup, warm it to no higher than 115 degrees Fahrenheit to maintain live enzymes. Season your food with warming spices—I'll discuss them later in this chapter.

Food Intolerances

One of the prime benefits of cleansing is learning how your body reacts to changes in your food. For many people I work with, this is an aha! moment. When they make the profound connection between what they eat and how they feel, their entire life changes.

This often occurs during a cleanse, after removing inflammatory foods and beginning to eat more whole foods with higher nutritional value. Energy rises, thinking becomes clearer, and moods lift. One client said to me, "I was driving down the road this morning, and I started laughing for no reason—for the sheer joy of feeling great."

Many people go through a detoxification phase when they begin a cleanse. They feel worse at first. You may experience aches, pains, headaches, and overall lethargy for several days. This is a sign that you're detoxing, and these symptoms will pass. Adding more cooked food or animal protein will slow the detox but make the process more comfortable. Stick to the cleanse protocol as much as possible, but follow your instincts and adjust your diet as needed.

If you haven't yet discovered whether you have intolerance to a food or food group, now is an opportune time to explore this possibility. Approaching this in a systematic fashion right after a cleanse will give you valuable insights into how the foods you suspect of being troublemakers affect you both in the short term and over time. This can provide useful information as you continue to discover and enjoy your individual Nutritional Style.

For a long time, I'd had a sense that dairy was a problem food for me. As a child, I got sick after eating my first ice cream sundae, but it took many years for me to realize that I got sick not from too much sugar and the excitement of the experience but from the milk in the ice cream. As an adult, I loved Parmesan cheese too much to acknowledge I had an intolerance to dairy. Parmesan was my condiment of choice for years, and while I knew it made me retain water and bloat, I was, in fact, addicted to the stuff. I ate other cheese here and there as appetizers, and enjoyed the occasional yogurt, but I never realized that my daily shake of Parmesan on salads or veggies was enough to keep me congested, with blocked sinuses susceptible to infection.

When I finally got real about giving up dairy, it changed my life. I left behind migraines, bloat, and the debilitating illnesses that I described at the start of this book.

You, too, can discover whether your system is intolerant to any foods, or if you should omit a food group from now on. Here's how to know: If you haven't already been on a cleanse, give up one common inflammatory food group completely for two to three weeks. For the experiment to work, you mustn't consume any variation on the foods or have even a taste of them during this phase. After your break from the food or food group, choose a day for reintroduction. If you did a full cleanse, add in only one food group at a time. If you're testing for a single intolerance, say dairy, on this day only reintroduce dairy products (even if you've given up some other food group as well). You can test for another food group in a week.

Enjoy several dairy products that day, enough to stimulate a reaction. This might include milk and cheese (but make sure the cheese doesn't contain gluten if you've given that up, too). Monitor

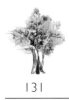

When I finally got real about giving up dairy, it changed my life.

how you feel during and after eating, later that evening, and through the next day. Signs of intolerance vary, but may include stomach pains, diarrhea, gas, bloating, nausea, headaches, lethargy, excessive mucus, and more.

If any of these signals appear, your body is talking to you. Congratulations. You've established the connection. You've learned to tune in and you now have power over your health and future.

If it turns out you are intolerant to dairy, or any of the other inflammatory food groups, the important point now is to accept it and act accordingly. Don't overthink this. Yes, you can go get lots of blood tests to look for allergies, but you don't really need them. The tests aren't as reliable as the elimination process—and the elimination process doesn't involve needles and doctor bills.

If you want to test for another food intolerance, say gluten, wait another week, while continuing a gluten-free lifestyle. Be sure to check the ingredients label on boxes, cans, jars, and bottles of any processed foods. Gluten is a hidden ingredient in many products. Watch out for ingredients such as artificial colors, artificial flavors, brewer's yeast, dextromaltose, emulsifiers, hydrolyzed protein or hydrolyzed wheat protein, malt or malt flavoring, and stabilizers. They can all contain gluten. Also, gluten is used in a lot of prescription and nonprescription drugs and in supplements. Again, check the labels and talk to your pharmacist.

RICK   Sugar and Joint Pain

One of my clients had been diagnosed with osteoarthritis in his late thirties. By the time Rick came to me in his forties, he had accepted the fact that arthritis ran in his family. His father had also suffered from it starting at an early age. Rick came to me not for his arthritis, however, but for help in cleaning up his diet and getting healthier overall. When we discussed his daily nutritional habits, we realized he ate a lot of sugary foods. My first suggestion to him was to give up the refined sugar. After just a few weeks without sugar, Rick noticed that his arthritis symptoms had disappeared.

A year later, months after we had stopped working together, Rick called me with some interesting news. He had been nervous before giving a presentation at work, so he had pulled a cookie off of a tray in the boardroom and ate it. Because he had gone without refined sugar for over a year, that cookie tasted really good, so he had another— and another, and another. On the drive home later that day, his knuckles were throbbing. He told me the pain was so bad he could barely hold the steering wheel.

Rick was easily able to pinpoint the problem: sugar = pain. His joints had responded to the sugary cookies he ate by becoming swollen and painful.

Choose a day to eat foods containing gluten. I recommend picking a day when you don't have any important business or social engagements. For breakfast, have a big piece of bread, a bagel, or some other form of wheat. Just don't eat anything that contains dairy (cereal with milk, for instance) or sugar (a doughnut, for instance) because that brings dairy and sugar into the picture. You want to test only your response to gluten, without any confusion from other foods you might be sensitive to.

Signs of gluten intolerance are pretty much the same as the ones for dairy. You might also feel itchy or have a skin rash; brain fog isn't uncommon. The important thing is to pay attention to your body and note how you feel.

This process can be repeated for soy, sugar, coffee, processed foods, and alcohol. My bet is that you'll find something surprising for at least one.

Once I discovered my food intolerances, I eliminated those foods and experienced a significant improvement in my health. My sinus issues cleared, and I haven't experienced a sinus infection in years. I rarely get sick or catch cold. I stopped getting migraines and seasonal allergies. My energy remains strong and steady without extreme highs or dips throughout the day. What you might personally discover about your own food intolerances could have a profound impact on the rest of your life.

On a holiday or special occasion, I sometimes eat a moderate amount of a food that I know is inflammatory to my system, but I do it consciously, fully aware that I may pay a price. I notice the impact if I have a cup of coffee (crazy energy), or eat some cheese (mucus in the back of my throat) or a piece of bread (stomach pains). It's easy to avoid these foods when I know the price of eating them.

DAWN | Unstalled Weight Loss

My client Dawn was having unexpected difficulty losing weight. Although she exercised and ate according to her Nutritional Style, her weight just wouldn't budge. She was getting discouraged. We went through her diet carefully to see if anything was new or different. Sure enough, her weight loss had stalled as soon as she returned to an old coffee habit. I asked her to try removing the coffee. She later happily reported that she had dropped several pounds starting right after she gave up the coffee again, and her weight loss was continuing. The coffee seems to have created an inflammatory effect that challenged her body, preventing it from releasing weight.

You might grieve when you discover intolerance to one of your favorite foods. It's often the foods we want the most that do the most harm. It might be possible for you to enjoy your forbidden foods in small amounts here and there, say on a major holiday or your birthday. Today, with so many gluten-free products, great tasting low-glycemic sweeteners, and more and more bakeries and food manufacturers making gluten-free, dairy-free treats, it's getting easier to enjoy delicious foods without having to suffer the side effects. More important, the longer I go without eating these foods, the less I crave or want them, or even really want a substitute for the real thing. Most of my clients feel the same way.

Your life doesn't have to be one of deprivation; moderation, adjustment, and discovery will let you continue to enjoy your food. Learn how to grocery shop and carve out time to prepare or order the foods that feed you well. Establish your health as a priority and stop eating what's in front of you just because it's available. Only you know what works for you. Tuning in to the foods you love and that love you back is an integral part of living your Nutritional Style.

When you do indulge, use caution. Given the addictive nature of some of these foods, it's easy to overdo it. All the unpleasant symptoms of eating inflammatory foods will come roaring back if you don't pay attention.

If you do consciously decide to indulge, make sure you choose the best quality you can find. If you're going to have a small scoop of ice cream, make it the top-end gourmet stuff in your very favorite flavor. I appreciate really good food, so I create and seek out new, easy recipes to keep me satisfied and happy, keeping the foods that trouble me out of my diet. You'll find a lot of great ideas posted on my website and blog at hollithompson.com.

Spice It Up

There's a reason we enjoy spiced pumpkin pie on Thanksgiving and crave savory stews and richer soups as we head into the chilly seasons. Our cultural traditions are steeped in centuries of a deep knowledge of how to use herbs for their medicinal benefits. For generations, the only medicines available came from the earth. People

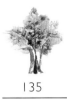

all over the world developed pharmacology traditions depending on their location and needs.

Herbalists believe that the earth has provided us with all the solutions we need, and in fact, many popular pharmaceuticals were created in laboratories to mimic plants found in nature. Aspirin, the original wonder drug, was created in a lab in 1897, but it was designed to mimic the active ingredient in willow bark, well-known in traditional folk medicine as a pain reliever. You can tap into these ancient ways by exploring how spices, herbs, and warming foods can help you feel satisfied and healthy.

The world of seasoning doesn't end with plain old salt and pepper. Herbs and spices provide a way to warm your body naturally in colder months. You can add health benefits to the dishes you prepare and also make cooking easy and fun by learning to use the warming spices of winter.

As a reminder that spices are for everyday use, my husband and I set up a condiment tray in our kitchen. We shopped for a variety of shakers and pots to hold our array of health-promoting spices. We store cayenne pepper in a shaker the way most people do for salt. We keep cinnamon in an old-school Parmesan shaker, and pots with chalkboard labels hold turmeric and ground ginger. Nutmeg is kept in a clear glass shaker, so we can see its brownish tone, and dried garlic is on view in a small Mason jar; another jar holds local honey. We keep a variety of salts on the condiment tray as well: Himalayan, Celtic, and a beautiful French gray.

> Some herbs have properties that boost immunity and protect you from viruses.

Favorite Herbs and Spices

In the fall, keep warming herbs in mind and ready to use in your kitchen. Some spices help with weight loss by creating heat, which revs your metabolism and improves circulation. Some herbs have properties that boost immunity and protect you from viruses. Others help soothe the stomach and digestion, fight inflammation, and even replace essential minerals. Check out this kitchen pharmacy for fall (it's good the rest of the year, too):

Cinnamon is at the top of my list for warming up and boosting the metabolism. It's antibacterial and good for immune support during cold and flu season. Try using it as a natural sweetener in smoothies, or sprinkled on roasted squash, carrots, and root vegetables.

Turmeric is a traditional ingredient in curry powder—it's what gives the mixture its yellow color. Turmeric is used around the globe as an anti-inflammatory. It's now becoming a popular means to help reduce inflammation and joint pain. Try adding turmeric to your savory stews or soups. It adds color and flavor and gives a home-made touch to the store-bought kind.

Ginger is one of my all-time favorite herbs and something that I eat almost daily. It's known for fighting nausea, which is why as a kid you may have been given ginger ale for an upset stomach. (Sadly, most ginger ales on the market today do not contain real ginger.) It's anti-inflammatory, relieves pain, and is warming to the body. I enjoy ginger in my green juice or smoothie. I always recommend fresh, organic ginger if you can find it. Your health food store probably has the organic kind; your grocery store has the regular kind. If you use nonorganic ginger, just be sure to peel it first. Dried ginger is great to keep on hand if you need it in a pinch, but the flavor isn't as fresh and pungent.

Nutmeg is an ingredient in pumpkin pie spice; where would we be without it at Thanksgiving? Like cinnamon, nutmeg is naturally sweet but nutty, and has antiviral properties as well. Try adding nutmeg to your vanilla smoothies for a taste similar to eggnog.

Cloves boost immunity, too, and are antiviral and anti-inflammatory. Cloves always remind me of my childhood; we used to push them into oranges to create a natural potpourri. (I still ask my son and his friends to do this every holiday.) Clove is wonderful added to stews for an exotic flavor. Use it sparingly, however; this spice is potent and a little goes a long way.

Garlic improves circulation and helps prevent blood clots, making it a natural choice for heart health. Garlic is an immune system powerhouse: It kills parasites, helps you heal, and is antibacterial and antiviral. And, of course, it adds a wonderful, pungent flavor to just about anything.

Cardamom is another spice commonly used in curry dishes. It's actually a member of the ginger family. It's an antioxidant, and contains potassium, magnesium, and other essential minerals. In addition to spicing up stews, try some cardamom along with cinnamon in drinking water once the weather turns cold for a warming, spicy effect.

Pumpkin and autumn squash

I love the way the farmers' market looks in the fall, when the harvest of orange, yellow, and deep tan squashes are piled high. Pumpkins bring back childhood memories of jack o' lanterns, but pumpkin is worth knowing about as a food, too. High in B vitamins that benefit your heart, pumpkin and its cousins offer bone support from potassium and cancer prevention from beta carotene (it's what makes them yellow or orange inside). Squash is a healthy carbohydrate that's really satisfying in a stick-to-your-ribs way.

Brussels sprouts

I crave brussels sprouts in the fall and winter. Luckily, my husband fancies himself a brussels sprouts chef—he roasts them in a large iron skillet, then tosses the browned sprouts with veggie broth and gluten-free pasta. (I prefer spaghetti squash pasta.) When you look at a brussels sprout, it looks a lot like a miniature cabbage. Actually, it is—brussels sprouts are members of the highly nutritious cruciferous vegetable family. These little vegetables offer two and a half times the daily requirement of vitamin K in just one cup. One serving also offers well over your daily requirement for vitamin C, which helps build your immunity in the fall for the winter cold and flu season. And they also contain folate, vitamin B6, and a good dose of fiber.

Pomegranate

Pomegranates were a symbol of fertility in ancient times. The many juicy red seeds were associated with fertility because of the way they're crammed into the fruit, but that's only because the ancients didn't know about antioxidants. Pomegranates are a great source of antioxidants such as cancer-fighting polyphenols. They're also an excellent source of vitamin C and potassium. I use pomegranate seeds to top salads during the holidays (so festive) and add

them to smoothies for the gorgeous red color and added vitamin C. The stumbling block? How to get those hundreds of little seeds out of their shell without turning you, and your white kitchen, pink. Try opening the pomegranate this way: Fill a large mixing bowl with cold water. Carve an X into the top of the pomegranate. Submerge the fruit in the water and insert your thumbs into the slits. Tear the fruit in pieces, then shake the seeds loose from the white membranes. The seeds will sink to the bottom of the bowl; pour the water and seeds into a strainer.

Cauliflower

One taste of my simple puréed cauliflower soup (see page 192) and you'll understand why this veggie is so darn super. Cauliflower is surprisingly high in immune-boosting vitamin C, plus it has plenty of vitamin K, folate, vitamin B6, and fiber to support smooth digestion. Raw foodies like to shred the florets to create vegan rice; flexible vegetarians love it mashed like a potato. Try roasting it with olive oil, too. Cauliflower has one more advantage: It stores very well in the fridge.

Dark leafy greens and kale

People who write about good nutrition are always talking about dark leafy greens (DLGs)— kale, spinach, collards, mustard greens, turnip greens, and others. That's because every one of the DLGs is a nutritional superfood, packed with vitamins, minerals, and fiber. One cup of cooked kale offers up 1,200 percent of your daily vitamin K and almost 600 percent of your daily vitamin A requirement. It also contains copper, manganese, calcium, potassium, and magnesium along with all that fiber. Superfood, indeed! The other greens are comparably super as well. Juice them, steam them, blend them, sauté them with lots of olive oil and garlic, rip them up into salads. Whatever you do, these veggies rock!

Sage has been used throughout history to preserve meats and treat respiratory ailments, so it's no wonder this tradition carried through the years as part of a Thanksgiving meal. Oniony-tasting sage is an appropriate choice for autumn cooking. This herb continues to grow even in cold weather, so it's often used as seasoning in the fall. Sage is what gives traditional turkey stuffing its rich flavor. Sage tea with honey and lemon juice is often used for coughs, sore throats, and laryngitis, and rumor has it some well-known opera singers use it, too. It's also used to clear brain fog and improve focus.

Fall is the harvest season and the time when farmers' markets and your local stores are bursting with variety, flavor, and phytonutrients. Fall's produce fortifies the body by being rich and varied; it's full of nourishing vitamins and bursting with nutrients. Enjoy a full array of superfood produce this fall to help prepare you for the dark and cold days of winter.

> Fall's produce fortifies the body by being rich and varied; it's full of nourishing vitamins and bursting with nutrients.

Juice or Smoothie?

Just as adding warming spices and herbs and seasonal vegetables help your digestion adjust to the cooler climate, the daily greens you eat may need to change as well. If you've spent the summer enjoying cooling, fresh vegetable and fruit juices, you may start to feel chilly as the fall days get cooler. One of the benefits of juiced vegetables is their quick and efficient absorption into your system, but when cool weather arrives, you might want and need to switch to smoothies instead.

Many people prefer a green smoothie in fall and winter because of the slower transit time in your digestion. The high-fiber content of a smoothie slows the absorption of nutrients, in contrast to the quick absorption of juice. A smoothie fills you up more and can feel more satisfying as the weather turns cool.

A vegetable or green smoothie consists of vegetables and a bit of fruit combined with a liquid, such as water or coconut water, in a high-speed blender. Blending retains the fiber of the vegetables and fruit. Because all the fiber is retained, smoothies help your digestion by allowing your body to absorb the beneficial nutrients more slowly.

I often get asked about the difference between smoothies and juices, and which method is better. The answer is, it depends. Both approaches have benefits. Your choice is determined by which one suits your Nutritional Style.

Juicing vegetables and fruits extracts the fiber, giving you a more watery liquid and nutrients that rush into your bloodstream. Juicing also uses a lot more produce—depending on the produce, juicing takes roughly five times more vegetables than a smoothie. Cucumbers, for example, produce a lot of juice because of their high water content, whereas kale produces a small amount of juice per leaf. This makes smoothies more cost-effective. On the other hand, because juicing uses so many vegetables, the amount of nutrients per serving is generally higher if you compare net weight to net weight.

The slower absorption of a vegetable smoothie can be beneficial to more delicate digestive systems. The additional fiber supports easier elimination, lowers cholesterol, and supports a healthy heart.

Vegetable smoothies are easier to make, especially in the morning rush—another reason to choose them in the busy months of fall. And most blenders are easy to clean with a quick rinse. Adding produce to water in the blender and turning it on takes just minutes, while the entire process of juicing—washing and prepping large amounts of vegetables, and cleaning the juicer afterward—can take fifteen to twenty minutes or even longer.

If you prefer juicing but have trouble sparing the time to make your own, look into purchasing pressed vegetable juices, either from your local health food store, pressed juice bar, or online (see the resources section at the back of this book). Pressed juices are the result of a laborious process that presses the ground pulp of the produce to extract juice. It's not a process that's easy to do at home, but pressed juice bars are popping up in a lot of cities. Make sure that the juice bar you frequent uses organic vegetables and fruits, and check the dates on the juices you purchase. Pressed juices last three days in the refrigerator, a bonus and a time-saver compared to home-juiced vegetables, which you should drink immediately. A new process has been developed to maintain pressed juices longer than three days, but I prefer the bright freshness of just pressed.

Some companies will deliver your juice to your home or office (see the resources section of this book). Stocking your refrigerator at home and at your office with fresh, pressed juice can save you loads

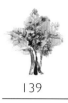

of time and energy. Because it takes a lot of time to make pressed juices, they can be expensive, but it may be worth the time saved.

I often switch to a high-fiber green smoothie in the fall months. The slower nutrient absorption rate seems to support my digestion as I adapt to colder weather. Because meals traditionally become more complex in the fall and winter, with more cooked and heavier foods, this time of year may call for additional fiber in the form of a smoothie for you as well.

Trust your taste buds and go with whichever form of liquid nutrition you prefer in taste and texture. Both have benefits—tune in to what you desire and what's easiest for your lifestyle.

Strengthening Immunity

Cold and flu season begins in the fall. If you have children, this is hard to forget because the school nurse sends out the first strep and flu warnings by early October. I start talking with my clients about immunity and defense against viruses and bacteria as early as August. As a precaution, I recommend taking probiotics in late August, so that the good bacteria will be in place by November when the cold and flu season arrives. This is particularly important if you work in a busy office, have children, or come into personal contact with a lot of people each day.

The key to immune system health is centered in the digestive tract, so a fall cleanse will help fortify your ability to fight off cold-weather germs. Adding a daily green smoothie or juice will provide high levels of antioxidants, an important piece of the puzzle. Adding warming herbs and spices will help, too, but many people still require additional immune support in fall and winter.

Adding immune-support supplements to your healthy eating regimen could make a big difference in the fall:

Probiotics are healthy bacteria necessary for a balanced digestive tract. Taking probiotic supplements helps you maintain a fully functioning digestive system and strengthens your immunity. Even if you feel healthy right now, your immunity might be compromised by factors such as stress, recent or frequent antibiotic use, and poor nutrition. Food sources of probiotics include naturally fermented foods such as sauerkraut, pickles, kombucha, and

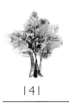

kimchi. Unflavored live-cultured yogurt also contains beneficial bacteria. If you can tolerate dairy, this is a good source. Watch out for commercial yogurt brands that claim to contain probiotics. They don't contain enough live bacteria to make them worth eating. Probiotics capsules are a good alternative. The health food store shelves here offer a wide range of choices. Look for capsules that contain the bacteria strain *Lactobacillus acidophilus* as well as other strains for broad protection. Since it's difficult to know which strains of bacteria you're lacking, I recommend switching your probiotic brand every few months. I prefer capsules that are stable at room temperature so that I can carry them with me when I travel. Many high-quality brands require refrigeration. If you purchase these, carry them straight home in an insulated bag and put them in the fridge right away.

Vitamin D. It may surprise you to learn that vitamin D boosts immunity by helping to activate and mobilize immune system cells that attack infections. The waning fall sun still can give you enough D to help increase your store right now, so soak up as much as possible before outside temperatures get too low. Have your vitamin D levels tested, and use a supplement if you find that you're low (check back to chapter seven for more on vitamin D).

Vitamin C. You need high levels of vitamin C to keep your immune system strong and help ward off illness as the fall flu season begins. Fortunately, this vitamin is abundant in whole food sources. Fall fruits, such as apples, pears, and citrus, are excellent sources; so are the wonderful fall squashes, such as butternut squash and pumpkin. You might not know, however, that red peppers and brussels sprouts are also excellent sources for C in the fall. Stress depletes vitamin C, so adding in more during this busy time of year makes sense. Your body doesn't store vitamin C, so if you feel you're not getting enough from your daily diet, consider supplements.

Vitamin B12, also called cobalamin, helps maintain a healthy nervous system and digestion. Because it's hard to absorb from food, and because your ability to absorb it diminishes with age, a surprising number of people are low or even deficient in this vitamin. Also, vitamin B12 is found only in animal foods. This means all vegans and most vegetarians need supplements, but even omnivores can run on the low side. Bonus: Many people report that taking vitamin B12 supplements helps boost their energy.

> Stress depletes vitamin C, so adding in more during this busy time of year makes sense.

Bach Flower Remedies

In the fall, as challenges like holiday planning, airline travel, back to school, and family commitments create additional stress on your immune system, additional support is helpful. A gentle approach that may work well for you—it helps many of my clients—is Bach flower remedies.

I've kept Bach flower remedies as a staple in my medicine cabinet for many years. Developed in the 1920s by Dr. Edward Bach, an English physician, these flower essences have been used by holistic health practitioners ever since. Dr. Bach identified 38 wildflower essences that he believed helped calm various negative emotions and, just as important, allow positive emotions to enter. Each flower is associated with a different emotion; taking a few drops of one flower essence or several in combination can help relieve the negative emotion.

Bach flower remedies are available as a kit containing small dropper bottles of each essence. I use the kit to create different combinations, depending on what's required. Bach flower essences are safe, although they sometimes contain a small amount of pure brandy as a preservative (you can get alcohol-free versions). They have no contraindications with any drugs or herbs. They can't cause harm, even if used in excess.

Bach flowers can be used to relieve focus and concentration issues, emotional eating, stress, anxiety, and more. They work well on adults and kids; they're even beneficial for dogs and horses!

Rescue Remedy is Bach's most famous blend, a combination of flower essences that is recommended for dealing with emergencies and stressful situations. The flower blend used in Rescue Remedy is great for helping you to relax and focus. It's available as drops, chewy pastilles, chewing gum, mouth spray, and in other formulations. I like to keep a bottle on my desk and add four drops to a glass of water three to four times a day. I recommend this approach to my clients. Some other ways to get the benefits of Rescue Remedy:

- Add four to five drops to your morning water bottle to sip while you drive the kids to school (better than coffee)!
- Place five drops under your tongue if you're experiencing acute stress or anxiety.

The flower blend used in Rescue Remedy is great for helping you to relax and focus.

- For pets, add four drops to the water bowl to help them adjust to a move or a household change. For pets that are injured or upset (from a thunderstorm, for instance), four drops under the tongue can be helpful.

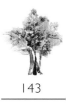
Fall Movement Style

With shorter days, waning sunlight hours, chilly mornings, and colder evenings, fall can be a challenging time to maintain a fitness routine. It's also probably the most important time of year to do it.

The holidays are coming, and if you have children in the household, the craziness begins in October. You need all the strength, flexibility, and metabolism-burning power possible right now, so keep moving. If your fitness routine diminishes now, it'll be more challenging to pick it up in January, when the holidays are over and it's freezing outside.

Indian summer can bring glorious days of colorful foliage and an ideal climate for being outdoors. Hiking in a park or getting outdoors for apple picking can connect you with the season and keep you active in a fun way. Take advantage of the local scenery, make a plan to go for a long walk with friends over the weekend, and reward yourself with a healthy brunch.

I continue to exercise outside until it gets too cold. In fall I put on layers of fleece and determination and get out into the fresh air as much as I can stand, knowing how much more energy I'll have and how much better I'll feel if I keep up my routine.

It gets dark earlier, so exercising at the end of the day isn't as appealing as it was in summer. The new priority is to get home at dark and snuggle with your honey or kids, or make a nice cozy dinner. Try switching your workout time to the morning, or take an exercise break midday. Allow time to soak up a few more rays of vitamin D-loaded sunshine, too.

Now is the time to make a fall exercise plan—before you lose the sunshine. Layer a jacket over your running clothes and stay outdoors, or head to the gym you joined ages ago and discover its new fitness classes. Convenience is the key this time of year. Keep your fall fitness routine close to home, and make it easy to eliminate all excuses. Consistency is imperative, so even if you only have time for a 20-minute workout, do it. You'll be happy and feel a sense of accomplishment.

Plan ahead, and realize you might feel discouraged on day three as your muscles rebel and your schedule hasn't caught up with you yet. Allow time to adjust to the new routine. You may need a week or two to learn to love your new fitness style, and a full month for it to become a habit that your body craves.

The best part is that when everyone else feels regret at dropping their fitness this December because they got too busy, you'll be on your game, and more productive, too.

Fall Beauty Style

Fall is a complex time for beauty, as your skin and hair react in different ways to the sudden change in weather. Some people get oily skin and breakouts. After a summer of drying sun and heat, your oil glands are still pumping and doing their job, and haven't caught up to the change in weather. Others complain of dry skin, their body's reaction to the onset of cooler weather. Many get a mixture of both, or combination skin. My friend Robin says, "I can't tell if my skin is dry or oily right now; it seems to be both!"

Your hair might be feeling the same way—scorched from the summer heat and sun exposure, and ready for a new cut; or oily at the scalp, as you adjust to less heat. This could be the time for a great new look and hairstyle, but either way, I think you'll love my do-it-yourself beauty remedies for fall.

Ancient Indian hair secret
Rosie owns a small hair salon near where I live, and one warm day in early fall, I told her about how dry my hair had gotten from swimming in the ocean. I had beach hair, but without the sexy, soft drape that I wanted. Instead of recommending one of her salon products, she offered to massage my head with almond oil.

Rosie claimed that almond oil is wonderful for blondes, but she loved what it did for her long, thick, glossy dark hair, adding that she massages almond oil into her children's scalps, and believes that it's great for the brain. She says that in her native India, they use it on the aging to help them retain memory function.

When I mentioned this story to my friend Lena, a natural blonde, later that day, we agreed to buy some right away. Lena and I decided that anything that gives you a healthier brain and silky hair as well is worth trying!

Quick tips for breakouts and dandruff

As the autumn air gets dryer and you spend more time indoors, skin blemishes and dandruff can start to appear. I like to avoid the harsh chemicals found in many blemish treatments and dandruff shampoos in favor of more natural remedies. Lemon juice is an astringent and a drying agent that can help with skin breakouts. Dab some with a cotton swab onto pimples to help dry and eliminate them. Tea tree oil, also known as melaleuca, comes from a type of myrtle plant native to Australia. It's antibacterial, antifungal, and antiviral; when dabbed on a breakout, it helps to dry the eruption fast. Tea tree oil also solves dandruff problems. Add a few drops to your regular shampoo and massage into your scalp, or mix tea tree oil with jojoba oil for a pre-shampoo treatment.

Almond Oil Hair Massage

Ingredients:

2 to 3 tbsp pure almond oil

Preparation: Working over the sink, pour a small amount of almond oil into your hands. Gently massage the oil into your scalp by separating sections in your hair. Let it set under a shower cap, or wrap your head in a warm towel. Leave the oil in for as long as possible, overnight if you can. The following day, wash with your normal shampoo and condition lightly to detangle if necessary. Style as usual.

Spicy Fall Body Scrub

Ingredients:

1 tsp local honey
1/4 c olive oil
1 c organic raw sugar or organic brown sugar
15 drops of cinnamon essential oil

If you work on your tan during the summer months, early fall can mean spotty, uneven skin as you lose your tan and shed dead cells, leaving your skin looking dull and lackluster. This body scrub helps to even out your skin tone and exfoliate dead skin cells; also, it smells heavenly. Cinnamon adds a warming scent to this sweet answer for smooth arms and legs.

Preparation: Add oil to the honey in a small bowl and blend with a small whisk. Add in the sugar and cinnamon essential oil and blend well.

This recipe makes enough for four to six uses. I store my scrubs in a glass wick jar container at room temperature.

Apply the scrub in the shower or tub. Rub gently in circular motions on dry skin. Pay extra attention to dry patches—knees, elbows, and wherever you notice uneven skin. Rinse with water. Be careful not to slip and make sure to remove the olive oil residue afterward to keep the shower or tub safe.

Ingredients:

1 tbsp raw oatmeal
2 tsp honey
1 tsp water or lemon juice

Oatmeal and Honey Mask

This mask for oily skin smells delicious enough to eat, and will help minimize post-summer breakouts. You can make it with lemon juice instead of water for added acne-fighting and astringent properties.

One of my clients is a young model and swears by this mask, preferring it to store-bought ones. She started using this before shoots for extra refining and to soften her pores.

Preparation: Grind the oats in a coffee grinder to a fine powder. In a small bowl, mix the ground oats with the honey and water or lemon juice. Apply the mask to the entire face, with the exception of the eye area. Allow the mask to sit for 10 to 20 minutes. Remove gently with a soft washcloth and warm water. This gets messy, so be sure to do it over the sink.

Ingredients:

1/2 avocado
1/4 c raw honey

Moisturizing Mask for Dry Skin

Dry skin needs something that will moisturize it naturally, without chemicals that can worsen the problem. Avocado is the answer. Avocado is a great source of healthy omega-3 fatty acids that moisturize you from the inside out. When you apply avocado to your skin, it helps build a soft, silky appearance. Mixing the avocado with honey gives you added benefits—honey has antibacterial and anti-inflammatory properties that help clean and protect your skin.

Preparation: Mash the avocado in a small bowl and mix well with the honey. Apply the mixture to your face with a brush and allow it to set for 10 minutes. Rinse.

I view my holistic health practices in the fall as an investment. If I take care of myself now, I'll have a happier holiday season and a healthier winter. That means my family will, too, because when Mama's happy, everybody's happy, right? The big message for autumn is: Don't drop the ball just because you're busy. We're all busy. You deserve to carve out time to keep your Nutritional Style on track, move that body, and pamper your skin. While you're at it, find time for some fun adventures outdoors to clear your head and lift your spirits. Winter's coming.

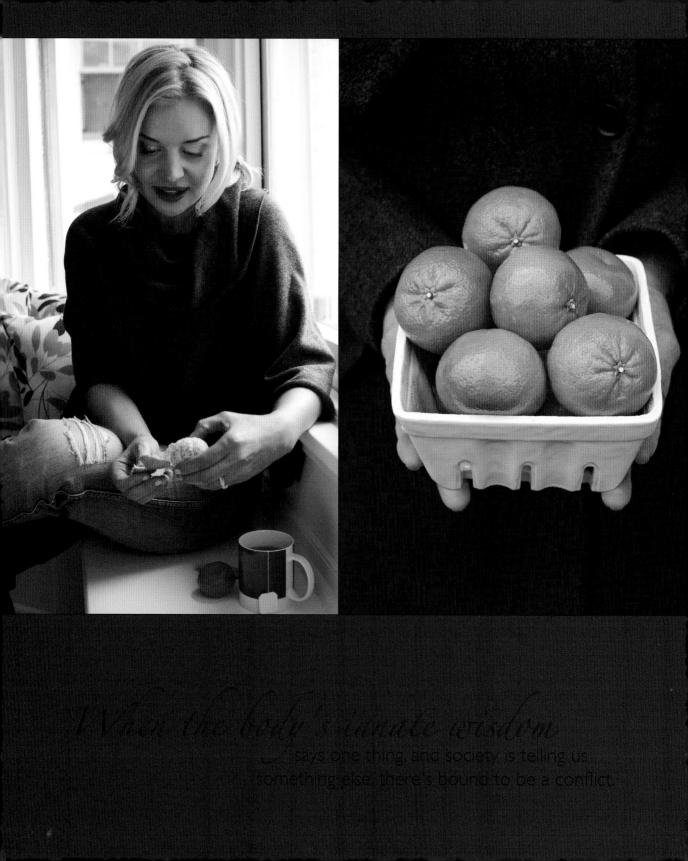

When the body's innate wisdom says one thing, and society is telling us something else, there's bound to be a conflict.

Winter Warmth

The glamour of the holiday season intoxicates as the world becomes red, green, and crazy with anticipation. You prepare, and shop, and wait for those special days with family and friends. Kids become impatient, counting the days to Christmas or Hanukkah, while you struggle to buy gifts, decorate the house, and plan outfits, dinners, and parties—maybe even look forward to a special night out for New Year's.

You might struggle with your nutrition during this time of year: party trays overflow with fatty, starchy appetizers, and open bars tempt you to have that extra glass of wine or cocktail, luring you away from your best-laid nutrition plans. A little bit here, and a whole lot there, and before you know it you might want to switch out your chic party dress or tux for a Santa suit.

While challenging at times, the holidays can be a joyous season to connect, have fun, and share the love. It all depends on your approach. In this chapter, you'll learn how to make the holidays a time of full hearts and skinny waistlines. We can give new meaning to surviving the holidays.

The New Year offers a chance for a fresh start, yet, our best intentions often dim after only a week or two. The dark days of winter seem to get even colder and shorter, and by February, you feel tired or even sad.

Both nature and history have predetermined that everything slows down in winter, in one way or another. We're biologically programmed to rest and conserve energy this time of year. Learning how to use this to your advantage will be the key to maintaining a healthy lifestyle.

The cold and flu season might force you to slow down if your immune system is weak, so I'm going to explain how to improve resistance to viruses and bacteria when the colder weather brings activities indoors. This is a wonderful time of year to fortify your body through nutrition. We'll dig deeper into some key strategies and important supplements that you'll want to remember all year long.

Winter can be a time of warm and graceful living, as your Nutritional Style flows with the season and all it offers: friends and deep connections, followed by quiet, solitude, and rest. You want to be ready to launch into action when spring arrives, even if it seems as if it will never come.

Ready to join me? Let's make this winter the best one yet for your ultimate health, productivity, and love of life.

The Holidays

When it comes to the holiday season, you have a choice—get carried away, falling victim to the media's timetable of events and the Hollywood version of what this time of year is supposed to look like, or not. You may choose to overspend, shop 'til you drop, bake homemade cookies for everyone you know, decorate a live tree with imported ornaments, host your entire family for a very long week, and cook the perfect goose with all the trimmings. You may decide that your kids and friends must receive the perfect gifts or that you must send a stylish holiday card with the perfect family photo. You may pressure yourself to get every other detail just so, right down to perfect holiday collars with jingle bells attached for your cats.

If you choose this route, chances are that you will end up exhausted, and if you're not careful, sick in bed by New Year's, collapsed under the weight of December's self-imposed burdens.

That was my story. I put the Holli in holi-day. It was my time of year. I did it all, and I spent several Januaries paying the price. Exhaustion, bloating, weight gain, depression, sadness—I had all these symptoms and more, and some years it took me months to recover. Being sick almost always forced me to give up my fitness routine, and my skin would turn a sickly shade of pale. I'd wrap myself in layers of black fleece and shuffle around in sheepskin boots. It was hard to get myself excited or enthusiastic about anything. Those were tough winters.

While I tried to justify it as simple fatigue, the truth was that my health had been compromised. I had lost track of my good nutrition, self-care, and nurturing habits. At the root of this were many complex health challenges, ranging from food intolerances to hormone imbalances due to pregnancy. Even so, I didn't have the knowledge or support I needed to know what to do, or how I could have avoided the traps. Since then, I have done the hard work and figured out what was getting me down. Now I share that knowledge.

I've helped hundreds of women discover how to live the lives they want during the holidays and throughout the year.

Surviving the Party Season

I've been through a lot of holiday parties—corporate, office, friends, and at home. It is possible to survive and even thrive through the party season—just follow these tips.

Eat first. I teach my clients that the best way to avoid a nutrition problem is to prepare and not leave things to chance. Counting on your holiday office party to serve healthy food won't always work, so be prepared. Eat something before the party begins to keep your blood sugar even and help you keep your resolve. If you walk into the party feeling hungry, you'll end up having that extra cookie, or driving too many crackers into the gooey dip. Instead, eat a healthy protein at your desk or before you leave the house. The snack will stabilize your blood sugar and improve your personal staying power. Almonds, walnuts, nut butter on celery, a few bites of animal protein, or a Nutritional Style smoothie all are great options.

Choose whole foods. If you can manage to eat only or mostly whole foods when you go out, you'll be ahead of the game the entire holiday season. Whole foods are foods with just one ingredient, such as celery, nuts, carrots, salmon, salad, and so on. That means avoid anything baked, goopy, creamy, oily, cheesy, or fatty, especially if you don't know the ingredients. If you have to compromise, choose something that's high in protein to sustain you, like hummus or goat cheese.

Multiple holiday buffets can be both your salvation and your downfall. The buffet will hopefully have green salad and some sort of vegetables and a protein, along with more tempting offerings. Choose the smallest plate you can and fill it full of whatever whole foods, like salad, veggies, and poached salmon, you can find. If you want to, treat yourself to a taste or maybe a small portion of something you don't usually eat, such as buttery mashed potatoes or gooey crab dip. You'll get to enjoy your favorite holiday treats without going too far off track. Ditto for the dessert tray—choose something that's a special holiday treat, the sort of thing that comes around only at this time of year, like a sliver of Yule log cake (my

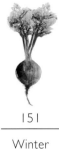

Whole foods are foods with just one ingredient, such as celery, nuts, carrots, salmon, salad, and so on.

personal favorite—I make sure to enjoy this on Christmas Day each year). Have the smallest possible portion.

Drink water. Water is just as important right now as it was back in the summer. It's just that now, in the winter, your body may not be urging you to drink, mostly because you don't feel hot. Between the colder temperatures and spending so much time indoors, many people forget to hydrate properly. But dry air from heating systems and long days out shopping or running errands require that you drink your water; otherwise, you'll face dry skin, hunger, and lower energy. Don't be that person! Remember to tote your water bottle along, buy some wherever you go if necessary (recycle the bottle), and drink a glass or two before meals or snacks. At parties, be the one who orders a sparkling water with lots of lime first, then, if you still want it, enjoy a cocktail or glass of wine. But then again . . .

Limit alcohol. Holiday parties highlight alcohol—from wine and cocktails, to eggnog with rum, to champagne, alcohol is the centerpiece of many holiday get-togethers. Too much alcohol can have some unwelcome side effects. Puffy eyes, dull skin, weight gain, a bloated appearance, and a tired look are all the after-effects of over-imbibing. Your energy levels suffer, too, as will your brain's capacity for clear, focused thinking.

Try alternating sparkling water with wine or a cocktail, or enjoy sparkling water with just a splash of wine or vodka. (If you can, make your own drink—bartenders have a tendency to give you full-strength drinks even when you ask for something lighter.) Or decide not to drink at all, and look forward to feeling fantastic the next morning. Today, many health-conscious people drink very moderately or not at all; you won't stand out as a party pooper.

I often pass on the alcohol during the holiday season, knowing that if I indulge at every party, I'll feel awful by New Year's. I celebrate on New Year's Eve with a glass of champagne, but often I feel so good without it, I don't want any.

Carry snacks. Just because your days are busier and filled with rushing around, don't take that as a reason to skip eating. You may not have time to sit down to breakfast or lunch, but you still need to keep your energy up and your mind sharp. Stock healthy snacks in your handbag, desk drawer, car console, and wherever else you're likely to find yourself feeling hungry. Smart choices include organic

> Enjoy what's in your mouth; savor the flavors, even if it's a trail mix that you've been snacking on for three days.

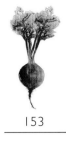

protein bars, snack bags of almonds and dried berries, or a pressed green juice.

Dress for nutrition success. Getting dressed for a special holiday party? However gorgeous, don't choose the loose silky top or the smoking jacket that covers everything. Opt instead for the fitted dress that makes you look like a star, or the narrow capris that reveal your waistline. You'll make healthier choices because you'll naturally become more body-conscious and aware of what you're eating.

One of my clients, Jen, calls this a sneaky, mean trick, but she loves it. She once was the queen of comfort, and in her first coaching session she described how she shrouded herself in loose black tops, dresses, and jackets in order to look thinner. What she didn't realize was that this was allowing her to eat without thinking because her clothing was hiding her tummy, and expanding with it. Dressing this way allowed her to rationalize that she'd begin to eat right tomorrow, but tomorrow never came.

Once Jen came to terms with her body weight and shape and dressed for it in a more flattering way, including slipping on the Spanx, she began to not only eat less but also feel better about herself. She looked thinner and felt fabulous, and she didn't add ten pounds to her petite frame that holiday season by snacking the night away.

Dine in slow motion. No matter how much rushing around you do this winter, establish this rule for any time you eat, even if it's on the go. Chew your food in slow motion, and think about what you're eating. Enjoy what's in your mouth; savor the flavors, even if it's a trail mix that you've been snacking on for three days. It's delicious, it's nourishing, and you're taking care of yourself. Allow the food to become a pasty liquid in your mouth before you swallow.

Chewing mindfully will assist in digestion, as your mouth sends a signal to your stomach, alerting it that food is on the way. You'll assimilate more nutrients from your food, and enjoy it more.

How full are you?

When you sit down to a meal, or to a plate of food from a holiday buffet, evaluate your hunger on a scale of one to ten. If one is famished and ten is as stuffed as a Thanksgiving turkey, evaluate how full you become as you eat. It takes 20 minutes for your brain to realize how satisfied you are, so stop when you feel you've hit five on the hunger scale, meaning satisfied but not stuffed. By the time your brain catches up, you'll be happy you did.

Exercise

Many people skip out on exercise during the holidays, but this is the worst thing you can do. You may not see the difference in your body right away, but you will feel it in your energy levels and focus. You need the emotional benefits of movement to help you deal with holiday stress. Exercise keeps anxiety at bay, helps you sleep, and keeps your moods on an even keel. Even if you shorten your routine a little or really have to skip a day, don't forget to move in some way, almost every day.

This might feel impossible in the midst of the frenzy of holiday shopping or a snowstorm that ties you indoors, but you'll feel better with some easy sit-ups, push-ups, and a few good dance moves to your playlist.

Share the love

During this giving time, remember those less fortunate than you. Giving money, gifts, or food to charities that sponsor families in need is a gracious way to keep your inner balance and demonstrate gratitude for all you have. If you can't afford to spend or give money, donating your time is just as meaningful.

Recovering from the Holidays

I love the holidays. And I love holiday meals. I want to celebrate with family, and friends who are like family, and enjoy good food, guilt free.

That's what holidays are for. So, even as you follow the tips I just gave you, ease up and enjoy! And then get back on track, starting the very next day. Here's how:

Drink water. Hydrating after a big meal will boost your metabolism and keep your body humming along. That's important, since you ate more than usual the day before—and maybe had more alcohol than usual, too. More water will increase your energy and make you feel clear-headed. Spice up a big pitcher of water (or several water bottles to take with you) with some cinnamon sticks or lemon slices, and sip throughout the day.

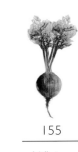

Have a green smoothie. You especially need to get your greens and phytonutrients today. A green smoothie will help balance your body and help you cleanse the inflammatory, rich foods from the day prior. The fiber will clean your digestion and help with elimination.

Eat protein. High-quality, easy-to-digest protein will support your metabolism and give you energy. Leftover turkey is easy, but stay away from the leftover stuffing. Instead, have your turkey on a big bed of greens (more fiber and phytonutrients). Quinoa is another great choice. It cooks quickly, so you can make a batch and enjoy it warm for breakfast with almond milk and goji berries. Later on, have it as pilaf, mixing in the leftover veggies.

Eat root vegetables. Seasonal root veggies are sweet, high in fiber, and satisfying, especially if you're avoiding carbs like leftover stuffing and dessert today. Roast sweet potatoes, squash, onions, carrots, and beets for a savory and sweet filling meal (or snack).

Move. Walk, stroll, skip; do something to help your body digest the big meal you enjoyed yesterday. Activity will help your digestion move things along and boost your metabolism. You'll burn your holiday meal pronto!

Winter Nutrition

> On the first of January, the year is brand-new, and so are you.

When the holidays end and January begins, most people get busy with their New Year's resolutions. To begin a diet and work-out regimen, particularly to lose the weight gained during the holidays, is the most common resolution. Believe me, I know. January is my busiest time as a health coach. Many people contact me then for help transforming their resolutions into a new and improved version of themselves by shedding pounds and getting healthy.

On the first of January, the year is brand-new, and so are you. All things seem possible coming off the holiday high, and yet for most, the quest is over a few weeks into January. Perhaps a snowstorm or a horrible cold stopped you. Maybe it was too chilly to rise at 6:00 a.m. to get on the treadmill, or the thought of green juice when what you really want is hot cereal turned you off. Or maybe the daily pressures of life when the days are dark and cold just got to you. Whatever happened, it has happened to many people. You, my friend, are not alone.

For centuries of human history we rested in winter. Our ancestors didn't have snow blowers or cars that defrost automatically. They didn't have the abundance of foods that we do, available 24/7 and shipped in from all over the planet. They were forced to conserve both food and energy during this time of year in order to survive. Their lives depended on resting, staying warm, and taking cover. They didn't have a choice.

In the twenty-first century we have almost infinite choices, but our bodies didn't get the memo. In the winter the body naturally wants to gain weight and slow down. It wants to sleep and prepare for spring, as it always did, when it needs all its strength and energy to plant fields and find food. When the body's innate wisdom says one thing, and New Year's resolutions and magazines are telling us something else, there's bound to be a conflict.

The challenge right now is that most people crave heavier, richer comfort food, like slow-cooked stews, chunky soups, pastas, chili, and grains, often prepared with cheese; and for Healthy Omnivores, more meat. These foods warm the body and provide a heavier, grounding energy. They also slow you down as nature intends in winter, so you might not feel as spry as you did back in June. The good news is if you learn to enjoy and embrace this time of year as part of the flow of life, it can bring a deep satisfaction without harming your health.

Enjoying more comfort foods is not a reason to abandon fitness or to eat whatever quantity of foods you desire, but it is a call to action to eat well and appropriately within your Nutritional Style. Stick with the foods that support your healthy lifestyle. Even as you do, you can still continue to lose weight in winter, though it's more challenging than at other times of year. Acknowledge this reality and allow your body's natural rhythm to play a role. Winter isn't the best time to pressure yourself by embarking on a weight-loss campaign. I generally advise my clients to just aim to maintain their weight during the holidays, which is an accomplishment in itself. I ask them to focus most of their efforts on staying healthy and keeping up their fitness during this time. Most of them who want to lose weight continue to do so, though perhaps more slowly.

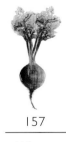

Winter Foods and Your Body's pH

You may find yourself craving more meat and animal proteins to fortify your body in colder weather, but venturing too far into a diet heavy in animal proteins isn't healthy for many reasons. Excessive meat consumption can lead to digestive disorders and has been linked to higher cancer rates, as well as heart disease.

Red meat is more difficult to digest, and has a longer transit time in your digestive system, so eat it only in moderation. A piece of fish, for example, passes through the digestive system much faster, while fruits can pass through quite quickly, within a few hours if eaten alone.

Animal proteins also make your body slightly acidic as they're digested. Your body likes to be very slightly on the alkaline side (the opposite of acidic), so eating foods that make you acidic means your body needs to neutralize them to maintain the right pH balance. (The pH number is a way to measure how acid or alkaline something is. A pH of 7 is neutral; below 7 is acidic, above 7 is alkaline.)

How to balance out your body's pH? It's surprisingly easy if you eat as you've been learning to throughout this book: green drinks, veggies, healthy whole grains, nuts, and beans are all on the alkaline side. Eat these foods in abundance and they will naturally neutralize the acidity from animal proteins and other foods. (Check the charts to the right for some acidic and alkaline foods.) A good way to keep the balance is to aim for 80 percent alkaline foods with the remaining 20 percent acidic. The challenge this time of year is to continue to eat vegetables and fruits and incorporate into your menu seasonal produce, like dark leafy greens, root vegetables, and winter squash, as well as fermented foods.

The pH theory is a bit controversial. Skeptics argue that the body is very good at maintaining its pH in the very narrow healthy range, no matter what you eat, except in extreme circumstances. That's probably true, but why not help your body out with that crucial task? There's no disputing that adding more vegetables while minimizing alcohol, meat, dairy, and other animal proteins is a healthier way to live. The positive results will reflect back in your overall health.

ALKALINE FOODS

Avocados
Beans and legumes
Fruits
Leafy green veggies
Millet
Nuts
Quinoa
Root vegetables
Sea vegetables
Wild rice

ACIDIC FOODS

Alcohol
Animal protein
Coffee and black tea
Dairy products
Refined grains, especially wheat, rice, and oats
Soda
Sugar of any kind (including honey)
Vinegar

Winter produce is less varied than seasonal produce the rest of the year, but these foods are grounding, just like the root vegetables that define the season. At this time of year, you need and crave warmth, with nourishment that will sustain you through the cold, dark days. This is the time to favor cooked or gently heated foods and support yourself with heavier dishes. Check out my favorite winter superfoods.

Sweet potato

This delicious, sweet, and starchy vegetable tastes like a guilty pleasure, but it's actually a queen among superfoods. It contains high levels of carotenoids, which your body needs to make vitamin A; one medium sweet potato provides the daily vitamin A requirement for children (and kids love them). Sweet potatoes are also high in vitamin C, vitamin B6, manganese, copper, and potassium. One baked sweet potato even provides 26 percent of your daily fiber requirement. To get the most from the carotenoids in sweet potatoes, enjoy them with a small amount of fat (extra-virgin olive oil or grass-fed butter, anyone?). The fat helps you absorb the carotenoids. For an easy and warming winter treat, slice a sweet potato into half-inch slices and steam them until they're just soft. Garnish with a drizzle of olive oil and sprinkle with cinnamon and nutmeg.

Cabbage

Cabbage is high in vitamin C, which is beneficial for immune support, and vitamin K, vitamin B6, manganese, potassium, iron, antioxidants such as polyphenols, and plenty of fiber. The nutrients in cabbage are at their highest when you eat it raw or only lightly cooked, but they're preserved even when cabbage is fermented, or made into old-fashioned sauerkraut the traditional way. I love cabbage in vegetable soups for a hearty fiber-rich stock; coleslaw is one of my favorite foods.

Beets

Beets contain potassium, magnesium, phosphorus, iron, and vitamins A, B, and C. They're also high in beta carotene, beta cyanine, folic acid, and fiber. They're cleansing to the liver and work to purify the blood. Naturally sweet, beets are delicious roasted, pickled, or shredded raw in salads. These gorgeous red beauties can stain your urine pink, a sign that your stomach acid is nice and low. Try yellow or orange beets, too, for a variety of phytonutrients.

Persimmon

One of my favorite sweet fruits, the persimmon is the official fruit of Japan. Its scientific name, *Diospyros*, means "fruit of the gods." My grandfather grew persimmons, so I learned to love them at an early age. They deserve superfood status thanks to high amounts of vitamins C and A, as well as beta carotene and heart-healthy lycopene. Persimmons also contain manganese, iron, and calcium. You can eat this fruit raw, but be sure that it's completely ripe—unripe persimmons are bitter and leave a fuzzy taste on your tongue. A good test for ripeness: Tug gently on the green stem. If it pops off easily, the fruit is ripe. Try persimmons as a fresh fruit, in a smoothie, and in salads.

Collards

If you live in the South, you know what a collard green is. A New Year's Day tradition says to eat hoppin' John, a dish made with collards and black-eyed peas, to bring luck for the coming years. This super dark leafy green is high in vitamins A, C, and K, plus has lots of B vitamins, calcium, manganese, iron, and even a nice shot of protein. Collards are perfect for winter because the hearty leaf needs to cook longer. They're delicious sautéed with onions and garlic, or added to stews or soups. Try using a large collard leaf as a wrap and filling it with hummus, avocado, and sprouts for a healthier alternative to bread.

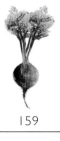

Supplementing Your Diet

I'm not a vitamin pusher. In fact, I hate taking pills. They make me gag. Over the years, I've consulted nutritionists who recommended supplements to the tune of adding hundreds of dollars to my monthly expenses. None of them ever gave me any food recommendations so that I could get what was in the supplements naturally instead. None ever recommended improving my diet, or even asked me how I was fueling myself; none ever made any connection between my food and my health issues. In their minds, what mattered was that I bought the supplements they recommended; they didn't even seem all that interested in whether I actually took them or if they helped. I used to have drawers and cupboards full of vitamins that someone promised would turn my health around, but full access to my own health came when I learned how to eat well.

When I became a health coach, I vowed that I would help my clients get their best nutrition from their food. No amount of supplements will ever replace a healthy diet. I do sometimes recommend supplements as needed—I'll discuss some later in this chapter. Used appropriately, the right ones can be very helpful and give you what you might not be able to get from your foods.

Winter is often the most challenging time of year for health. Cold and flu viruses are plentiful now, and we're sharing them with each other more because we're indoors together more, usually with the windows closed. Also, in the colder weather we need more energy to stay warm and comfortable. Add in how the lack of sunlight reduces our production of vitamin D and weakens our immune support, and supplementation can make sense.

Supplements are also needed more in winter because your food may not be as nutrient-rich as it is at other times of the year. The broccoli you buy in February, for instance, was probably grown in California or Mexico and spent a week in transit before you bought it—losing its nutrients the whole time. It's still got plenty of vitamin C and other good stuff, but not as much as the locally grown broccoli you bought in August. So, especially in the winter, you might want to be taking some extra vitamins and minerals—a daily multi-supplement is good insurance. You might also want to consider some other supplements that are particularly helpful for warding off winter woes. I've listed some of the most effective here, but use all supplements with caution. If you take any prescription drugs, have any chronic health problem, are pregnant or trying to get pregnant, for example, talk to a skilled health practitioner (not the clerk at the health food store) before taking any supplements.

Herbs for winter health

Elderberry. This herb is antiviral and an excellent choice to ward off colds. It warms the body and is sold as a tasty berry-flavored tablet or syrup, making it my top choice for travel and times when I feel rundown. I keep elderberry tablets in my travel tote for life on the go. My Swedish ancestors used elderberry as a health tonic, and syrups and jams made from this berry are popular in Scandinavia still. I recommend elderberry as a staple in your medicine cabinet for most of the winter. Try to find some elderberry jam while you're at it—it's the best.

Astragalus. In traditional Chinese medicine the root of this plant is used as a warming tonic to build resistance to diseases and to increase energy. This is a good herb to reach for if you require immune support—many herbalists recommend taking it at the first sign of a cold. My friend Dielle, an enlightened organic-farm owner, recommended this to me about a decade ago for a horrible cold I was fighting, and it's been in our medicine cabinet ever since. It's generally sold in capsule form.

Echinacea. The root of this plant, also known as purple cone-flower (a popular garden perennial), was used by Native Americans as a treatment for infections and snakebites. It's commonly used today to enhance the immune system and fight infection, especially for the common cold and upper respiratory issues. When my husband has a cold (rarely!), I like to give him echinacea in tincture form—he adds several drops to his morning juice, and puts several drops in every glass of water he drinks during the day. It's also available as tablets. Don't use echinacea if you have an immune system disorder, such as HIV/AIDS, multiple sclerosis, tuberculosis, or rheumatologic disease.

Vitamins and minerals

Although I believe in meeting our nutritional requirements with food, at times some people may need more support. Winter can be one of those times, especially if you're coping with additional stress

> Astragalus is a good herb to reach for if you require immune support—many herbalists recommend taking it at the first sign of a cold.

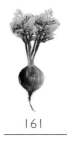

and health challenges, combined with less sunlight and vitamin D. I recommend using supplements derived from whole food sources if possible, and not chemically manufactured. Ask for whole food multivitamin brands at your local health food store.

Minerals are as essential to your overall health as breathing, and a lack of vital minerals can result in issues such as digestive absorption problems, bone density loss, muscle contractions, and brain malfunction. Although mineral supplements often are included with a multivitamin, sometimes you need more of some minerals than you can get from a multi-supplement. You might need some extra calcium, for instance, if you're showing early signs of osteoporosis; people with type 2 diabetes are often low on magnesium. In addition, excessive exercise, heavy sweating, stress, and aging all contribute to mineral loss. If you suspect you're low on important minerals, such as iron or magnesium, ask your doctor for a blood test to check.

B vitamins. The vitamin B complex has eight members. Each is a different but related vitamin, and each is equally important to your health. You need all the B vitamins for numerous body functions, such as supporting your brain and hormone balance, keeping your heart healthy, feeding healthy skin, nails, and hair, helping with digestion, and keeping your immune system working at peak levels. B vitamins often are included in a multivitamin, but the amount of each is usually below the recommended daily amount. The B vitamins in general are hard to absorb from your food, plus your body can't store them. Even if you have a good diet and take a multivitamin supplement, you might still need additional support, especially in the winter. Stress or illness can really deplete your B levels, so consider taking a B50 supplement, which contains all the Bs at half the recommended daily amount—you'll be getting the rest from your food and your multivitamin if you take one.

Vitamin B12 (cobalamin). This member of the B family is so crucial that I'm discussing it separately. You need vitamin B12 to keep your red blood cells healthy (a shortage causes anemia), to keep your immune system strong, and to keep your nerves healthy. A surprising number of people are deficient in vitamin B12. The amount of B12 in food is small to begin with and it's hard to absorb—and your ability to absorb it declines with age. Only animal foods contain vitamin B12, so if you're a strict vegetarian or vegan, you're not getting any from your diet and must take a supplement. I ask all my clients who don't eat animal foods to have their doctor do a blood test for B12 levels. The results often come back on the low side. When the client begins taking a B12 supplement containing 1,000 mcg, their blood test results improve and they feel more energetic.

Digestive enzymes. Your body naturally produces hundreds of different digestive enzymes that break down the various kinds of food in your intestines. Producing the right enzymes is a fair amount of work for your digestive system, so sometimes you want to give it a break. Plant foods that aren't heated to above 115 degrees Fahrenheit still contain their own natural enzymes. When you eat them, your body doesn't have to build any of its own enzymes to digest them. That's a major benefit of eating raw foods. Over the long term, your body has to do less work and can put its energy toward other things. This is the improved-energy bonus raw foodists enjoy. When food is cooked, your body must provide enzymes to break it down; for example, lipase for fats, lactase for dairy, protease for protein, amylase for carbohydrates, and so on.

Some people, for a variety of reasons, don't produce all the enzymes they need to break down a varied diet. Many adults no longer produce the enzyme lactase, for instance, which is needed to break down the lactose in milk and some dairy products. Other people may be slow producers of enzymes such as lipase, which is needed to break down dietary fat. Also, as we age our bodies are slower to make the right enzymes.

Taking supplemental digestive enzymes can help quite a bit. One of my clients, Lara, suffered from gas and bloating for years. We worked diligently on her diet and health, and she felt fantastic once she discovered and stayed within her Nutritional Style, but the gas and bloating were still there. The missing piece of her puzzle turned out to be digestive enzymes—the problem disappeared once she started taking them.

I recommend a broad-spectrum supplement that contains at least three plant-based enzymes, including protease, lipase, and amylase. Take one or two capsules about ten minutes before each meal; you'll probably notice a positive effect after a few days. Even if your digestion is usually iron-clad, I suggest taking digestive enzymes along when you're traveling. Your digestive system can take a few days to start making the right enzymes if you have a change in your diet or are eating a different cuisine.

Sleep for Ultimate Health

We're programmed to slow down during winter, just as our ancestors did for thousands of centuries before us. They rested and slept more in the cold, short days of winter not only because there wasn't much else to do, but because sleeping helped them to keep warm and conserve energy. We're no different—winter is when we seem to require the most sleep.

An integral part of our holistic health, sleep restores and repairs the body overnight. It allows organs to synchronize, muscles to rest, and the brain to process and store information from the day. Sleep deprivation can lead to memory loss, confusion, and an inability to make smart, or even safe, decisions. It can also have long-term effects on aging and appearance, creating wrinkles, eye bags, and a tired look.

Sleep deprivation also causes weight gain. Lack of sleep can throw off your hormones in ways that can lead to cravings for sugary and fatty foods and out-of-control eating. If you're sleep-deprived, your hormones might be influencing you without you even knowing it. Ghrelin, a hormone that tells your brain to eat, increases when you sleep poorly. Leptin, the hormone that helps you to slow down your eating when you're full, doesn't work as well when you miss sleep. Without the right hormonal signals, you'll keep on eating way beyond what you need.

Long-term sleep deprivation can lead to higher insulin levels, which impairs your ability to burn fat—you store it instead. And missing sleep, even as little as an hour, can create stress and make you over-secrete the stress hormones cortisol and adrenaline. High cortisol levels make the body not just store fat, but hold onto it tightly. When your cortisol levels are high, your body can't tap into your fat stores to burn them for energy. Cortisol also lowers serotonin, the feel-good brain chemical that helps you to stick to your well-intended eating plan. If you're tired all the time, you lose the resolve to stick to anything. Life becomes more difficult, leading to compulsive eating or even food bingeing. You also get cranky, have trouble remembering minor details, and can't concentrate well.

Lack of sleep leads to negative health and cognitive impacts, but it also influences your appearance—there's a reason it's called

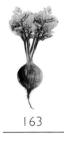

> An integral part of our holistic health, sleep restores and repairs the body overnight.

beauty sleep. When you don't sleep enough, it shows in your eyes: you might have reddened or bloodshot eyes, droopy eyelids, puffy eyes, and dark circles under your eyes. It also shows in your skin. Lack of sleep makes you look pale, wrinkly, and unhealthy; any skin blemishes stand out that much more. Lack of sleep might also make your skin age faster and slow down its ability to repair itself.

How much sleep do you need? Probably more than you're getting—just about everybody today, even babies, is sleep-deprived to some extent. Most people do best when they get seven to eight hours of sleep each night, but on average, American adults get less than seven. If this is sounding familiar, think about your waking time. Paradoxically, you might be a lot more productive if you spent less time on your computer and more time asleep.

With all these good reasons to get your sleep, especially this time of year, here are a few suggestions on how to fall asleep gently.

Magnesium. Among many other things it does in your body, magnesium helps you settle down to sleep at night. If you're on the low side for this essential mineral, you might have trouble falling asleep or staying asleep. A magnesium shortage can also be the underlying cause of restless legs syndrome, a disorder that makes you feel a powerful urge to move your legs, especially when you're lying down or resting. Needless to say, restless legs syndrome will keep you up at night. Magnesium supplements in the form of magnesium malate or magnesium citrate may help insomnia, but be cautious with them: they can also cause diarrhea. Keep your dose at no more than 350 mg, taken a couple of hours before you plan to go to sleep. A better approach is to eat foods high in magnesium a few hours before bedtime. Beans, nuts, whole grains, and dark leafy vegetables are all excellent sources. I've found that one of the unexpected benefits my clients report to me is that green drinks in the morning seem to help them sleep better that night, probably because they're getting more magnesium. They also have fewer headaches and migraines—this too may well be from the extra magnesium.

Lavender. The delightful aroma of lavender essential oil both relaxes and calms; it's well known for its soporific effects. Add a few drops of lavender oil to your evening bath or sprinkle a few drops on the shower floor before you turn on the water. Spray lavender on

> Spray lavender on your pillow or sheets, or diffuse some in your bedroom.

your pillow or sheets, or diffuse some in your bedroom. Put a drop on your wrists or on the bottom of your feet and between your toes for a restful, peaceful sleep. I keep lavender in my handbag for plane travel to use when I want to relax.

Herbal sleep teas. Herbs such as chamomile, passionflower, and lemon balm all promote droopy eyelids. Try them in the form of herbal teas or tinctures before bedtime—they can often make a big difference in your sleeping habits. Try them individually, make your own combinations, or purchase sleep tea or relaxation tea blends. Beware not to have them during the workday. I did that once by mistake and couldn't imagine why I suddenly needed a nap!

Limit caffeine. The opposite of a sleep aid, caffeine is the most common culprit behind sleepless nights. Try avoiding it after 1:00 p.m. or, if you turn out to be very sensitive to it, taking it out of your life altogether. I've seen this happen with several clients: They didn't want to believe their morning coffee could impair their sleep at 2:00 a.m., but after they cut out the coffee, their sleep improved.

Limit alcohol. Many of my clients come to me thinking that a glass of wine or some brandy in the evening helps them fall asleep. Because alcohol relaxes your muscles, it may actually put you to sleep, but you probably won't stay asleep. Alcohol causes disturbed sleep patterns that may wake you in the middle of the night and keep you from getting back to sleep. Eliminate all alcohol for at least four hours before bedtime and you may well see a big improvement in your sleep quality.

Turn off the screens. At least one hour before bedtime, turn off the screens and take out a good book (the printed kind). Studies show that those of us (guilty sometimes!) who get in bed with our laptops or tablets tend to get less sleep, and you know now the problems that can cause. Also, electronic screens, including TVs, give off a lot of blue light, which is damaging to your eyes. Tell the late-night hosts you'll catch them online the next day.

Winter Movement Style

Get up, even if you don't feel like it. Get out, even if it's tough. Click PLAY on that exercise video and move, even if you'd rather be in bed.

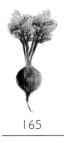

Winter can be the most challenging of times to stick to a fitness routine, beginning with the holidays and an over-booked schedule. Pile on snowstorms, cold, rain, and the gray skies of January and February, and you'd rather cozy up on the sofa with a hot chocolate for months on end.

Staying indoors and not exposing yourself to the cold means that your body doesn't need to work to stay warm or create extra body heat, so you'll miss out on some serious calorie burning. Being outdoors in the cold increases your calorie use; good to remember when you're tempted to skip your walk, and a great reason to get back to skiing or skating.

Some days, though, it's just impossible to venture out. Fortunately, video sites geared toward the at-home exerciser abound. Whether you prefer yoga, barre, cardio, Pilates, rowing, boot camps—you can have it. All you really need is a player and a screen.

Some online classes are offered though a live stream, which is attractive to those who love the intensity of a class. Others are pre-recorded and loaded onto a membership site, offering an unlimited number of views for a monthly fee. Still others offer live personal training, which is similar to a live experience, except you can maneuver how you appear in the camera for a more flattering view (downward dog, anyone?). YouTube is a great source of free exercise videos to follow at home. The range of choices is huge—you're bound to find an instructor or program that works for you.

For the more disciplined or less cold averse, a trip to the gym is still a great option, or hop onto a treadmill or exercise bike at home while you watch the morning shows. My choice is a portable rebounder, or mini-trampoline. For me, it's fun and energizing. I keep it in front of my desk, and take short jump breaks between clients, or bounce while watching my favorite cooking show. Rebounding is a good toner and builds core strength, while exercising you all over. It's also an effective way to stimulate your lymphatic system, which helps you to detox and supports immunity.

Whatever fitness style you choose, be sure to hang on to your routine this winter. Plan for it, try out several options, and commit to moving above all else.

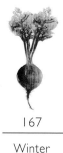

Winter Beauty Style

The winter season is full of beauty challenges, from stress, to cold air, to dry heat. Many people struggle with their appearance as a result. Your hair might be dry and have excess static electricity from blasts of heat coming out of the furnace. Your hands may develop flakey and chapped skin and your nails may break easily. Your skin might lose its rosy complexion, no matter how many green juices you drink, as a result of being indoors all day and breathing recycled office air.

Here's a winter roundup of do-it-yourself beauty products that will help you keep your healthy glow.

Winter Skin Scrub

This scrub uses sesame oil, which not only softens and penetrates dry skin, but also smells warm and toasty. Adding in the sweetness of sugar, the spicy aroma of cloves, and the zest of orange gives this a delicious aroma, but the secret ingredient is dried rose petals. Adding dried roses this time of year is my reminder that spring will come, even if it's below zero outside. This aromatic scrub is sure to lift your spirits.

This scrub is best used on semi-damp skin. Concentrate on dry and flakey areas, and go gently on or avoid tender areas. This is best used in the shower and rinsed off. Enjoy once or twice a week.

Preparation: Combine all ingredients in a bowl and mix gently. Store scrub in a glass jar or container.

Ingredients:

3/4 c organic raw sugar
1 tsp ground cloves
2 tsp grated orange zest
1½ c cold-pressed sesame oil
2 tbsp dried rose petals

Epsom Salts and Lavender Soak

Epsom salts are mostly magnesium, and in the same way that magnesium relaxes you internally, it absorbs through your skin as well to relax your weary body. Epsom salts are inexpensive and readily available. This bath works to relieve stress and help you sleep, too.

Preparation: Add Epsom salts to a warm bath under running water; then add the essential oil of your choice.

Ingredients:

2 c Epsom salts
20 drops lavender essential oil (or 20 drops peppermint oil or wild orange oil if you want an energy lift)

Ingredients:

1 c 100% aloe vera gel
10 drops frankincense oil

Aloe and Frankincense Moisturizer

Many years ago I met a woman who had the most gorgeous skin I'd ever seen. It wasn't just that it was wrinkle-free; it was flawless and naturally soft and clear. I couldn't resist asking for her secret, something that I don't normally do.

Her reaction and gentle smile told me she'd been asked this many times. She told me her mother had raised her to apply aloe vera gel to her skin, twice a day, and it was all she'd ever used.

I knew she was sincere, because I'd seen the wonder of aloe's works on myself at a young age after a terrible sunburn, but she confirmed it for me. You can use aloe straight as a moisturizer that doesn't have a greasy feel. For additional healing and anti-aging benefits, incorporate the warm and spicy aroma of frankincense.

Frankincense is known for improving skin tone and conditioning the skin. It helps prevent wrinkles and even heals scars. It's a luxury oil, but because it works great in small doses, a bottle goes a long way. My client Shane loves this oil as a wrinkle fighter. She combines it with aloe gel or coconut oil and smoothes the blend into her skin several times a week.

Preparation: Gently shake or stir to combine and store in a glass bottle or jar. Massage a small amount onto your face and body to soften and rejuvenate your skin.

Ingredients:

1 ripe avocado
1 tbsp raw honey
2 tbsp olive oil

Avocado-Honey Hair Mask

Due to dry indoor heat and cold winds, even the healthiest hair can begin to look dull in the winter. Mix up your own moisture-infusing hair mask with three ingredients already in your Nutritional Style cupboard. This mask is a delicious solution to dry, flyaway hair.

Massage the mixture through your hair; comb it through with a wide-tooth comb if you need to. (This is best done over the sink to avoid a mess.) Wrap your hair in a hot towel, straight from the dryer, and allow this treatment to penetrate your hair for at least 20 minutes. Rinse and shampoo as usual.

Preparation: In a small bowl, mash together the avocado, honey, and olive oil until the mixture is creamy.

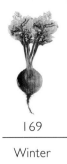

The quiet days of winter are a wonderful time to focus on you and what makes you happy and healthy. Maybe it's your chance to finally work with a health coach, take a cooking class, read a good book on nutrition, or join in on a group cleanse. Take advantage of this time, when your body naturally wants to rest more, and spend more time close to home and hearth. Give yourself permission to learn and experiment to discover your Nutritional Style.

You've learned dozens of new ideas and ways to take better care of yourself in this book. Not every idea is right for you, but some will really resonate. Work them into your life slowly and steadily, and notice how small changes can have big payoffs. Think of all these ideas, suggestions, tips, recipes, and must-dos as pasta (gluten-free, of course) that's been boiling on the stove. When you toss a few strands at the refrigerator, one or two will stick right away. Go with those.

Try the new ideas that seem to speak to you. The ones that give you an ah-ha moment. The suggestions that excite you and call you to try them, right away. Your body and your intuition know best. Save the rest for now and circle back in a couple of weeks for more. That's how I've worked with my clients, over time, and that's how I transformed my health years ago.

Go slowly, practice forgiveness, and don't aim for perfect. Keep moving forward, and when something becomes part of your lifestyle, you're ready for more.

My goal is to give you recipes that will spark your imagination and show you how healthy eating is also enjoyable eating.

CHAPTER TEN

Recipes for Your Nutritional Style

Most of the cooking that I do is quick and simple, because life is busy, right? I have a thriving business, a family, and a farm full of rescued pets. I don't always have time to put on a cute apron and design elaborate dinners. I like dishes that are easy to make, use lots of fresh ingredients, and fit the season. Cool salads in summer, warm soups in winter, and most important, dishes that match my Nutritional Style. The recipes in this chapter are organized by season. They're all appropriate for Healthy Omnivores and Flexible Vegetarians. Modern Vegans will find that most of the recipes are appropriate for them, too. My goal is to give you recipes that will spark your imagination and show you how healthy eating is also enjoyable eating.

In the seasonal chapters of this book I listed my favorite seasonal superfoods—the spring greens that help you detoxify after a long winter, summer's cooling veggies and fruits, autumn's warming foods, and the satisfying foods we crave in winter. In this chapter, I start off by listing my favorite year-round superfoods. These are foods that are good for you no matter when you eat them. Keep them on hand in your pantry for adding extra nutrition and flavor to your dishes.

The recipes in this chapter are mostly the easy, everyday solutions to feeding my family and me with love and fresh veggies. Some are my personal favorites, some are my son's faves, many are my husband's favorites. And some have been contributed by my wonderful friends and colleagues. I hope you'll find recipes here that will become your own favorites.

One of my main goals with this book is to persuade you that eating according to the season is the healthiest and most natural approach to your nutrition. When you eat seasonally, you'll begin to crave more seasonal foods and will feel more in touch with what your body needs and wants. In the growing season, discover your local farmers' markets and farm stands. That's where you'll find the freshest and most seasonal produce—and you'll be supporting your local farmers as well. In the off season, look for winter farmers' markets. Locally grown produce such as carrots, squash, potatoes, and an array of root vegetables will be available.

Welcome to my kitchen! I'm so glad you're here!

YEAR-ROUND SUPERFOODS

A superfood is any food that's particularly good for you for lots of good reasons, such as being high in fiber, or a rich source of antioxidants, or loaded with folate. Plus, a superfood tastes good, is fairly easy to find in a supermarket or health food store (or online!), and doesn't need a lot of complicated preparation. Asking me to choose my favorite superfoods is like asking me to choose my favorite pet. It's impossible, but here's my best try. I had to narrow this list to just my top year-round favorites—otherwise it would be pages long! Forgive me, maple syrup and cherries!

Apples

Apples are the first item on my year-round superfoods list, and not because they come first alphabetically or because they're so convenient to eat. There's just nothing as delicious as biting into a sweet, crispy apple! The outstanding nutrition that comes with it is just a bonus. Apples are rich in health-giving polyphenols and antioxidants. Eat them whole for the most benefit—the peel is a great source of pectin, a soluble fiber that helps keep you regular and may help lower your cholesterol. One medium apple has about 10 mg of vitamin C, 5 grams of fiber, and 240 mg of potassium. Apples are also a good source of the B vitamins riboflavin, thiamin, and vitamin B6. If you're lucky enough to live in apple country, modern storage techniques mean that locally grown apples are available throughout the year. If you can't buy the local kind, you're still sure to find half a dozen or more varieties at any food store. If you prefer your apples in juice form, look for refrigerated fresh apple cider. Apple juice—the kind sold in bottles and juice boxes—is sometimes sweetened with added high-fructose corn syrup.

Avocado

I refused to eat avocados for years, telling myself that they were fattening because of their high oil content. What I didn't know then was that our bodies need fat for healthy skin, hair, and digestion and to facilitate weight loss. Avocados provide plenty of healthy monounsaturated fat, as well as potassium, vitamins C, K, folate, and B6. They're also an excellent source of fiber and vegetable protein. These mildly nutty and scrumptious fruits (yes, an avocado is a fruit—technically, it's a large berry) are now part of my diet on most days. I enjoy them mashed with lemon juice, onion, cayenne pepper, and Celtic sea salt, on top of a green salad, or spread onto whole-grain gluten-free bread for an occasional treat. Avocados with a rough-textured skin are the Hass variety; Florida avocados have a smooth, shiny skin. Both are equally nutritious and delicious.

Bee pollen

Bee pollen contains twenty-two amino acids, including the eight essential ones, and an assortment of enzymes that benefit our health. There are also dozens of vitamins and minerals in bee pollen, along with natural hormones and valuable fatty acids. Taking bee pollen in small doses can help with seasonal allergies and allow your body to develop immunity to offending pollen allergens. This seems to work best if you take a daily dose for a few weeks before the allergy season for you kicks in. Try a spoonful of bee pollen in your smoothies for a superfood boost.

Berries

I surrender. I can't choose, so please don't make me. Blueberries, goji berries, golden berries, elderberries, raspberries, cranberries, mulberries . . . I want them all. Berries provide high levels of antioxidants, plenty of fiber, lots of vitamin C, and are powerhouses of nutrition in other ways as well. Goji berries, for instance, are rich in vitamin A. They're native to China, where they're used in traditional Chinese medicine to treat a wide range of conditions, including diabetes and high blood pressure. (These powerful berries may also interact with some prescription medications, including blood thinners and drugs for diabetes and high blood pressure.) Blueberries are the classic American berry. They're amazingly high in vitamin C and rank the highest of any berry in immunity-boosting antioxidants. Elderberries are immunity super-foods, too. I rely on elderberry syrup and homemade elderberry jam to keep my family healthy. (You'll find elderberry tablets in my carry-on luggage, always, to help me fend off germs while traveling.) Dried mulberries and golden berries are favorites among nutrition gurus and raw foodies. Like all berries, they're high in vitamin C and off the charts when it comes to antioxidant power. You'll almost always find them in my trail mix.

Chia seeds

As a kid, I always wondered how those tiny seeds got stuck inside my chia pet. As an adult, I now know chia seeds become gelatinous when wet, swelling up like tiny tapioca pellets. We love homemade chia pudding in our house (see the recipe on page 184); my son has grown up enjoying it for breakfast. Chia seeds are anti-inflammatory and loaded with heart-healthy omega-3 fatty acids. That makes them especially good for brain health. Chia seeds also contain fiber, calcium, and magnesium, along with plant protein. Many people find them helpful for stabilizing blood sugar. Try adding some chia seeds to your smoothies or sprinkling them into a salad for extra energy and stamina. This is one you've got to try.

Cacao powder and unsweetened cacao nibs

Cacao powder, more commonly known as cocoa, is made by grinding cacao nuts (the source of chocolate). Cacao nibs are small pieces of the nut. Natural cacao is actually bitter in taste. It's only trans-formed into the chocolate you know and love by adding lots of a sweetener, generally white processed sugar. I love cacao, but I don't want white sugar in my diet. Instead, I use natural sweeteners such as coco-nut sugar, stevia, or even maple syrup to create healthy treats with cacao powder or nibs. Cacao is loaded with natural chemicals called flavonoids, which act as powerful antioxidants—cacao is a superfood for your cardiovascular system. It also contains zinc, potassium, calcium, and magnesium. I add cacao powder to my smoothie on days when I need an energy boost. Among the ancient Mayans and Aztecs of cacao's home in Central America, the pods were used as a form of currency. My cacao treats are so good I could probably use them as currency, too (see the recipe on page 188).

Coconut oil

What would I do without this healthy oil in my life? I use coconut oil on my skin as a moisturizer, on my hair as a conditioner, and I even rub it into my slate kitchen countertops to keep them looking good. I give my dogs the occasional teaspoon, too. On your skin, coconut oil is antifungal and antibacte-rial. For years, coconut oil had a bad rap for being a saturated fat and supposedly bad for your heart. In fact, research shows that coconut oil can be a heart-healthy fat! It's true that highly processed coconut oil, the kind used in junky snack foods and baked goods, probably isn't good for you—its nutritional value has been stripped away. However, organic, pure coconut oil stimulates the production of good cholesterol and helps thyroid health. It also helps stabilize blood sugar. Use coconut oil as you would any vegetable oil. It's great for sautéing vegetables, frying eggs, and as a way to add healthy fat to your smoothie. Coconut oil is safe to use for high-heat cooking. It's loved by Healthy Omnivores and Modern Vegans alike.

Extra-virgin olive oil (EVOO)

I promised my parents I'd include EVOO in my superfoods list; it's their claim to longevity and looking good, and the good news is this kitchen staple absolutely deserves to be here. EVOO is a healthy fat and a staple of the Mediterranean diet. Use EVOO for salad dressings or to finish any dish in a healthy way. Extra-virgin olive oil is more stable than plain olive oil and provides anti-inflammatory benefits. It's high in oleic acid and monounsaturated fats. Look for brands that are cold-pressed. This method extracts the oil from the olive without added chemicals or heat. To be sure you're getting the finest and purest olive oil possible, check the label for quality seals from the country of origin.

Flaxseeds

If taste plays a part in selecting a superfood (and for me, it does), flaxseeds more than earn their spot on my list. These nutty tasting little seeds are best when ground so your body can absorb their superb nutritional offerings. Whole flaxseeds can pass through your digestion untouched. Flax seeds offer anti-inflammatory and antioxidant protection. They're a great source of lignans, or natural phytoestrogens. Some women approaching or in menopause find a daily dose of flaxseeds gives them some relief from symptoms such as hot flashes. Lignans may also help protect against breast cancer and against the plaques that can block your arteries and cause a heart attack. Flaxseeds are a great source of healthy omega-3 fatty acids—1 tablespoon of ground flaxseed has nearly 2 grams of omega-3s. They also contain a lot of soluble fiber in the form of mucilage, so they're great for intestinal support and keeping you regular. Flaxseeds contain copper, manganese, and magnesium; they're also an excellent source of vitamin E. Try adding a tablespoon or two of ground flax to your morning smoothie. Sprinkle it on salads or vegetables, or add it to your baked muffins or raw treats. Flaxseeds can go rancid quickly because of their high oil content. Buy them fresh and keep them refrigerated until you're ready to use them. If possible, grind the seeds freshly yourself. Flaxseed oil doesn't contain the fiber of the seeds, but it has most of the other benefits. Don't cook with flaxseed oil, however—heat destroys its benefits. Use this light, nutty-tasting oil to add flavor, much as you would use butter.

Green powder

Generally made with spirulina (a type of algae), chlorella (another type of algae), wheatgrass, or a mixture of one or more, green powders are rich in chlorophyll and detoxifying enzymes. Use in moderate amounts (just a spoonful or two a day) as a dietary supplement, or add it to soups and stews for a nutritional boost. Be sure to choose only raw, organic brands.

Hemp seeds

These small, round seeds have a delicate flavor; many people say they taste like pine nuts. They're a favorite source of plant protein among Modern Vegans and Flexible Vegetarians because they contain all the amino acids (the building blocks of protein) you need for good health. I use hemp seeds to top my salads and blend them into smoothies for a protein boost. Hemp seeds are also an excellent plant source of omega-3 fatty acids. Because Modern Vegans and many Flexible Vegetarians don't get omega-3s from fish, hemp seeds are a great alternative. Hemp seeds also help your memory. Make this little superfood a part of your daily diet now and thank yourself in about 20 years.

Kombu

A type of kelp widely used in Japanese cooking, kombu adds richness and depth to soups and stews. When kombu is added to the soaking and cooking liquid for dried beans, it cuts down on gassiness. It's sold in dried sheets. Break off a piece to use and store the rest in an air-tight container in the pantry. You can find kombu in any health food store or Asian grocery.

Kombucha

Forget the wine, pass me a kombucha at cocktail hour. Kombucha is a fermented drink made from a culture of bacteria and yeast in sweetened black tea. It originated in northern China many centuries ago and made its way to us through Russia. Kombucha tea is sweet, with a bit of fizz and a hint of vinegar. It's very high in B vitamins. Because kombucha tea contains beneficial bacteria from the fermentation process, it helps to stimulate the immune system and improve your digestion. Kombucha has become so popular that many commercial brands are now available. If you can find a homemade variety from a local producer, try it! If you have a DIY streak, you can brew your own kombucha. The cultures are easy to buy online. The only other ingredients you need are sugar, water, and black tea. Check food52.com, one of my favorite websites, to order your own brewing kit.

Maca powder

Made from the root of a plant that grows high in the Andes of Peru, maca powder is a good source of carbohydrates—nutritionally, maca is similar to wheat, but without the gluten. Maca is also a good source of protein, amino acids, and fiber, and it's high in calcium and potassium. In alternative medicine, maca is recommended as an energy booster and a way to increase stamina. Add a spoonful or two of the powder to your smoothies and green drinks. It's almost tasteless.

Nutritional yeast

This superfood was popular back in the 1960s and '70s. It's now enjoying a revival from its hippie days. Nutritional yeast is high in B vitamins, especially vitamin B12. This makes it popular with Flexible Vegetarians and Modern Vegans, because a diet with no animal foods is low in all the B vitamins and doesn't contain vitamin B12 at all. Nutritional yeast fills in the gap—but only if you buy a product that says it has the vitamin in it. Nutritional yeast is also a good source of protein and fiber. It has a cheesy flavor and is especially popular in creative raw food cuisine. I love it sprinkled on popcorn. You'll also often find it on top of my salads or garnishing roasted cauliflower florets.

Nuts

Why would you think I could choose just one? All nuts are a great source of omega-3 fatty acids, vitamins, and minerals, to say nothing of fiber. Almonds are high in vitamin E and calcium, while walnuts boost brain health with the most omega-3s of any nut, along with potassium and magnesium. Cashews contain oleic acid (like EVOO) for heart health and offer magnesium for your bones and nervous system. I love creamy, organic, raw nut butters. They're great to spread on celery sticks, stir into your morning oatmeal, or blend into a smoothie. Add your nuts of choice to salads, millet pilafs, gluten-free granola, or just make your own snack mix with some of the super-berries you love. A note about peanuts: Technically, peanuts are legumes, or members of the pea family, and not nuts. For all practical purposes, however, use peanuts as you would any other nut. People who are allergic to peanuts may also be allergic to tree nuts.

Quinoa

Quinoa (pronounced KEEN wah) has become so popular in the past few years that we're creating a global shortage. This ancient food is often referred to as a grain, but it's actually the seed of a plant in the amaranth family. It's a staple food in the Andes region of South America, for a good reason. Its highly concentrated nutrient profile contains balanced protein and the full spectrum of essential amino acids. Quinoa is high in vitamin E and heart-healthy fats and is impressive in its overall phytonutrient profile, too. It's also a great source of calcium, making it a good choice for vegans and people who are lactose-intolerant. It offers lots of antioxidants that support overall vitality and health. Even better, quinoa is also gluten-free. This anti-inflammatory seed can be sprouted and eaten raw, or cooked much as rice is and enjoyed in a variety of ways. Warm it for breakfast with fresh almond milk, cinnamon, nutmeg, and goji berries. Add vegetable broth, onions, and vegetables for a lunch or dinner pilaf. Or enjoy it mixed with kale and an EVOO vinaigrette for a satisfying salad.

Wild salmon

I hope that salmon continue to exist wild in Alaska forever, and remain free of the mercury that's so concerning in ocean-caught fish. Wild-caught Alaskan salmon (never the farmed kind) is a wonder food that provides an abundance of heart-healthy omega-3 fatty acids along with high-quality protein for you Healthy Omnivores. Wild salmon also offers vitamins B12 and D (both difficult to obtain from food), along with other B vitamins, magnesium, zinc, and iron. Salmon is quick and easy to prepare. It's delicious in all different ways—sautéed, baked, grilled, and even cured, as my Swedish friends do.

Sauerkraut

This year-round standby is always in my refrigerator. I take probiotics and recommend them to my clients, but naturally fermented raw sauerkraut is an excellent way to obtain healthy bacteria from a whole food. Fermented bacteria support your digestion and increase your immune health, especially important in cold and flu season. Sauerkraut is generally made from green cabbage, which is rich in fiber and vitamins A and C, but any fermented vegetable will provide benefits, so vary it up. And make sure you enjoy the sauerkraut juice when you're done. Oh yes, I do. I purchase my sauerkraut raw and fresh at a local health food store, but hope to make my own, any day now. It's easy to do. The Korean version of sauerkraut is called kimchi, a spicy combination of cabbage, ginger, hot red pepper, garlic, and scallions. It's highly addictive and all that garlic helps you make friends, fast. Kidding. Kimchi might call for peppermint essential oil in your pocket to keep your breath fresh, but it's amazing for your health.

Spring Recipes

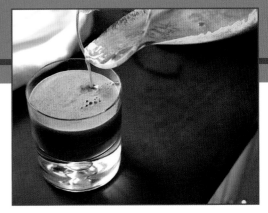

As the days begin to lengthen and warm up in spring, it's time to lighten up your diet. Ease out of your winter menu and sedentary lifestyle and take advantage of the tender produce and sweet baby greens that arrive with the season. Cleanse away winter's heavy menu with green juice and smoothies, asparagus soup, and the sweetness of fresh peas and early strawberries. The chickens are laying again, the salmon are running, and everyone is on the move. Are you?

Green Power Juice

This is my basic green juice recipe, the foundation drink for all Nutritional Styles. The greens are sweetened by adding fruit, and spiced with ginger. The base of the juice consists of light greens or veggies that contain a lot of water. Add in dark leafy greens, such as spinach, kale, chard, collards, or dandelion, for their nutrient value. Change them up according to your taste, what's fresh at the market, and to vary your nutrition. Ditto for herbs like cilantro. If you don't like it, try fresh parsley (preferably the flat leaf kind) or some other favorite fresh herb to add flavor, or just leave the herbs out. Instead of the apple, try a different sweet and juicy fruit, such as mango, pear, or pineapple. If you need to watch your sugar intake, leave the fruit out. The lemon juice can be swapped for lime, but one or the other is nonnegotiable for making your juice taste like green lemonade. Store the extra juice in a glass container in the fridge; use it within a few hours. This recipe is just your basic starting point. Your green juice is a work in progress, just like you. Feel free to improvise, adjust, and change. If you don't have a home juicer (yes, they're pricey), make this in a blender—it will come out as a delicious green smoothie.

Preparation: Rinse all the ingredients well. Add them to the juicer and run until the liquid is smooth. Makes about 32 ounces.

Ingredients:

- 2 cucumbers with skin (peel them if not organic)
- 3 stalks celery
- 2 c spinach
- 5 leaves chard or kale
- 1 bunch cilantro
- 1 Granny Smith apple
- 1 lemon with ends removed and rind on (remove rind if not organic)
- 1-inch piece of ginger (more if you prefer)

Ingredients:

1/2 c fresh strawberries,
    stems removed
1 tbsp hemp seeds
1 tsp chia seeds
1 tsp ground flaxseeds
1 tbsp raw coconut flakes
1 frozen banana
dash cinnamon
5 drops vanilla stevia
1 tsp vanilla extract
8 oz coconut water or water

Sweet Strawberry Banana Smoothie

Fresh, local, organic strawberries are completely different from the tasteless, jumbo-sized variety found year-round in the grocery store. Strawberries are among the most heavily sprayed and fertilized commercial crops. Avoid chemical and pesticide residue, support real farmers, and help the planet by buying only organic strawberries. This smoothie has flax, chia, and hemp seeds added for extra protein. Any or all can be left out if you don't have them on hand. This smoothie is my go-to choice for a mid-afternoon boost on a hot day—I keep peeled and frozen bananas in the freezer.

Preparation: Combine all the ingredients in a blender and process at high speed until smooth. Makes 12 ounces.

Ingredients:

1/2 c pine nuts
1/4 c nutritional yeast
    flakes
1/2 tsp sea salt

Vegan Parmesan

This is a delicious solution to the Parmesan problem for Modern Vegans or anyone who avoids dairy. The nutritional yeast is what gives this recipe its cheesy flavor. It stores for weeks in the refrigerator in a sealed glass container. Keep it on hand and use as you would real Parmesan cheese—it's wonderful on pasta. It's also great on popcorn, added to soup, and in a salad. Nutritional yeast is deactivated yeast, usually sold in the form of flakes or a powder. It's one of my year-round superfoods (see page 172). Look for it in any natural foods store. I prefer a brand that has added vitamin B12, a nutrient that Modern Vegans must be sure to get.

Preparation: Combine the pine nuts, nutritional yeast, and sea salt in a food processor. Pulse until well mixed but slightly crumbly, about 10 to 12 times. Store in the refrigerator. Makes 1/2 cup.

Ingredients:

1 c raw almonds, soaked
    overnight in water to
    cover in the refrigerator
3 c filtered water
2 medjool dates, pitted
2 tsp vanilla extract

DIY Almond Milk

Store-bought almond milk often contains added sugar along with additives that you might prefer not to eat. Making your own dairy-free almond milk is super easy. It took me a while to get into the DIY habit, but once you taste how delicious this is and how easy it is to make, you'll be hooked. You can flavor your almond milk with raw cacao and add a few more dates to create a homemade chocolate milk that rivals any store-bought brand. Just ask my son. You'll need a nut-milk bag, sprouts bag, or cheesecloth bag to make this—you can easily buy one at any health food store or kitchen supply store.

Preparation: Combine the soaked almonds and the water in a blender. Process on high speed until smooth. Pour the mixture into the nut-milk bag. Gently squeeze the milk through the bag into a bowl. Discard the almond skins left in the bag. Return the milk to the blender and add the dates and vanilla. Process on high speed until smooth. Store the milk in a glass container in the refrigerator. It keeps well for several days. Makes 4 c.

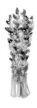

Banana Nut Ice Cream

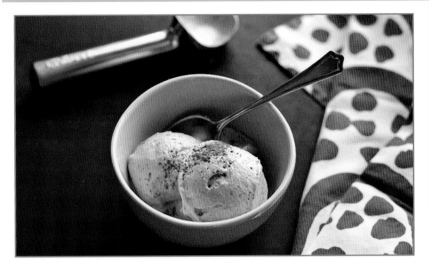

Ingredients:

1 banana
1/4 c raw pecans
1/4 c raw almonds
1 tsp vanilla extract
1 packet stevia to taste
    (you can also use 1/4 c
    coconut sugar)
1 tsp coconut extract
1 tbsp raw shredded
    coconut
2 c ice
splash almond milk

Healthy Omnivores, get ready! This recipe will make you forget you ever knew those two guys from Vermont who use dairy in their treats. In Virginia, where I live, the spring weather turns hot long before summer arrives. I make this for my family almost every night in hot weather and I don't mind a bit.

Preparation: Combine all the ingredients in your blender. Process at slow speed to begin; if needed, add a splash or two of almond milk to get the blending started. Gradually increase the blender speed and process until smooth. Serve immediately, topped if desired by Pantry Granola (see the recipe on page 191). Makes 4 servings.

Quinoa and Bean Salad with Mango

Ingredients:

This dish is a favorite at potlucks. Last spring I made it for a tailgate party we co-hosted for our local point-to-point. That's a horse race with jumps over grass—it's an exciting spectator sport, even more so if you're riding. This salad became an instant tradition. The leftovers (if there are any) are even better the next day. Make the salad at least a few hours or even a day in advance and let the flavors blend in the refrigerator. This is a great meal for Flexible Vegetarians and Modern Vegans, an all-in-one meal with a delicious combination of flavors.

1 mango, peeled and cubed
1 red bell pepper, seeded
    and diced
1 c chopped scallions
1 c chopped cilantro
    (optional—not everybody
    loves this herb as I do)
2 tbsp red wine vinegar
1 tbsp mirin
2 tbsp grape seed oil
2 c cooked quinoa
15 oz cooked black beans
sea salt to taste

Preparation: Combine all the ingredients in a large serving bowl and mix gently. Season to taste with sea salt. Makes 6 servings.

Ingredients:

2 tsp olive oil

1 bunch asparagus, roughly
  chopped (snap off the
  tough bottom parts first)

1 medium onion, roughly
  chopped

2 celery stalks, roughly
  chopped

pinch dried thyme or a few
  sprigs fresh thyme leaves

3½ c organic vegetable
  broth

1/2 avocado, peeled and
  thinly sliced

sea salt to taste

black pepper to taste

Creamy Asparagus Soup

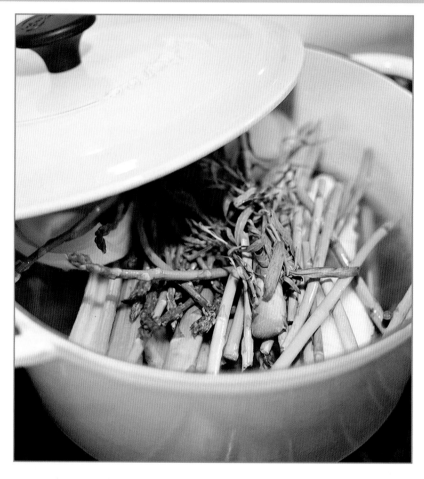

Asparagus season is in the early spring, when there's often still a chill in the air. This warm and creamy asparagus soup is great for a comforting lunch or casual supper. Modern Vegans will swear it contains dairy, but it doesn't. The vegetables cook down and become quite creamy when they're blended. This easy recipe is a spring stand-by in our home.

Preparation: Heat the oil in a large, heavy pot or Dutch oven. Add the asparagus, onion, celery, and thyme and cook, stirring often, until the vegetables are softened. Add the broth and simmer for 20 to 30 minutes. Transfer the soup to a blender or food processor, in batches if necessary, and process until smooth. Alternatively, use an immersion blender to puree the soup in the pot. If you used the blender or food processor, return the soup to the pot. Season to taste with sea salt and pepper. Serve garnished with the avocado slices. Makes 4 servings.

Honey-Glazed Carrots

Honey-glazed carrots are a favorite at our farm, especially in the spring when the carrots are small and tender. I especially love using heirloom carrot varieties with colors ranging from deep ruby reds to vibrant orange and sunny yellow. Adding local raw honey is not only sweetly delicious, but can help with seasonal pollen allergies. Try taking a teaspoon a day of locally produced honey, beginning sometime in late February or before allergy season begins where you live. Because it comes from where you live, the honey contains small amounts of pollen that match the kind that makes you sneeze. By eating some every day, you may desensitize yourself and have fewer allergy symptoms.

Preparation: Preheat oven to 350°F. Place the whole carrots into a deep baking dish. Drizzle them with the olive oil and stir until the carrots are completely coated. Add the honey and season to taste with sea salt and pepper. Mix gently again to coat the carrots. Bake until the carrots are just tender, approximately 45 minutes to 1 hour. Makes 4 servings.

Ingredients:

2 lbs carrots, tops trimmed
6 tbsp olive oil
1/2 c local, raw honey
sea salt to taste
black pepper to taste

Spinach Pesto with Sautéed Chicken

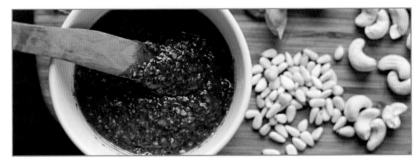

Pesto is traditionally made with basil, pine nuts, and Parmesan cheese. In this variation, spinach, one of the earliest spring greens, is added to the basil to boost the nutritional quotient with more calcium, iron, and phyto-nutrients. The lemon juice adds a fresh flavor. Sheep cheese stands in for the Parmesan. You can use the pesto to top fish, vegetables, pasta, or grains. Try stirring a spoonful or two into vegetable soup. Store any extra in an air-tight container in the refrigerator. To keep the top from blackening, pour a thin layer of olive oil over it.

Preparation: Combine the spinach, basil, garlic, and pine nuts in a food processor or blender. Process, gradually adding the olive oil and lemon juice. Add more olive oil if the pesto seems dry. Season with sea salt and cayenne pepper to taste. To sauté the chicken breasts, sprinkle them with sea salt and black pepper to taste. Heat the coconut or grape seed oil in a large, nonstick skillet over medium-high heat. Add the chicken breast halves and cook 6 minutes on each side or until the juices run clear when the chicken is pierced with a fork. Top each chicken piece with 1 heaping tbsp of the pesto. Makes 4 servings.

Ingredients:

Pesto:
2 c baby spinach leaves
1 c basil leaves
3 garlic cloves
1/4 c pine nuts
1/2 c extra-virgin olive oil
3 tbsp lemon juice
sea salt to taste
cayenne pepper to taste
1/4 c grated raw sheep
  cheese
Sautéed chicken:
4 organic chicken breast
  halves
sea salt to taste
black pepper to taste
1 tbsp coconut oil or
  grape seed oil

Summer Recipes

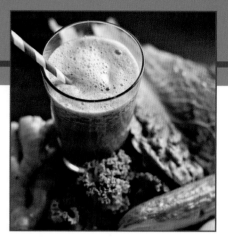

Summer brings the finest hot weather produce, including peaches, berries, tomatoes, and flavorful herbs. Savor the variety and the freshness. Summer's colorful produce wants to cool you down and keep you energized, so you can tend to your garden and your busy lifestyle. You're surrounded in summer with an abundance of fresh veggies—eat more raw is your motto now.

Ingredients:

- 1/2 head romaine lettuce, cut into thirds
- 1 cucumber, thickly sliced
- 1 cup dark leafy greens (such as kale, spinach, or chard), torn into pieces
- 1 lemon, sliced (peel it if not organic)
- 1/4 avocado, peeled and sliced
- 2 c coconut water
- 2 c water (if needed)
- stevia to taste (optional)
- 1-inch piece fresh ginger (optional)
- 1 banana (optional)

Green Goodness Smoothie

This smoothie is one of my personal favorites for vibrant energy. I love the sweet and sour effect from using coconut water and a lemon, but you can substitute plain water for coconut water, too. If you prefer a sweeter drink, add some of the optional ingredients. This smoothie is a fantastic way to start your day, flooding your cells with bright and happy phytonutrients. It's also alkalizing to your system, an important counterbalance if you're eating too much animal protein and processed foods. I say this serves two, but I usually keep it all to myself! Store the extra in a glass container in the refrigerator and drink it later that day.

Preparation: Combine the romaine lettuce, cucumber, dark leafy greens, lemon slices, avocado, and coconut water in a blender. Add stevia, ginger, and/or banana if desired. Process on high speed until smooth. If the mixture is too thick for your taste, stir in up to 2 c of water to thin. Makes approximately 60 ounces.

Ingredients:

- 2 tbsp extra-virgin olive oil
- 4 6-oz salmon fillets
- 3 tbsp fresh lemon juice
- 1/4 tsp garlic powder
- sea salt to taste
- black pepper to taste
- 1 to 2 tbsp stone-ground mustard
- 2 tbsp fresh dill, chopped

Roasted Salmon with Mustard and Dill

This recipe was contributed by Frank Lipman, MD, founder of Eleven Eleven Wellness Center in New York City. In addition to being an expert on nutrition and cleansing, Dr. Lipman is the author of *Revive: Stop Feeling Spent and Start Living Again*. His salmon dish is perfect for Healthy Omnivores and for Flexible Vegetarians who feel the need for some animal protein. The fresh dill gives it a wonderful spring flavor.

Preparation: Preheat oven to 375°F. Spread 1 tbsp olive oil in the bottom of a baking dish. Place the salmon fillets skin-side down in the dish and sprinkle them with the lemon juice. Drizzle the remaining 1 tbsp olive oil over them. Sprinkle the fillets with the garlic powder, sea salt, and black pepper. Spread the mustard evenly over the salmon and sprinkle with the dill. Bake until the salmon is fork tender and flakes easily, about 10 minutes. Makes 4 servings.

Chia Fresca

Here's my favorite DIY sports recovery drink, perfect for restoring your energy after a day in the sun. (Avoid store-bought sports drinks; they're loaded with added sugar and chemicals.) This drink is beneficial for boosting brain power, too. It'll help keep you sharp when you're in front of your computer all day. Chia seeds are one of my favorite superfoods. They're anti-inflammatory and very high in omega-3 fatty acids. They also contain protein, fiber, calcium, magnesium, copper, iron, and zinc. For this recipe, use whole chia seeds, not the ground kind. The whole seeds absorb up to ten times their weight in liquid and are readily digested by your body. If you make this with plain water instead of coconut water and want a sweeter drink, sweeten it to taste with some coconut sugar or a few drops of lemon stevia.

Preparation: Fill a 12-ounce glass with the coconut water or plain water. Add the chia seeds and stir well. Squeeze the lemon or lime juice into the mixture and stir well again. Sweeten to taste if using plain water. Let stand for 10 minutes before drinking. Makes 1 serving.

Ingredients:

8 to 10 oz coconut water or plain water
1 tsp chia seeds
1/4 fresh lemon or 1/2 lime
1 tsp coconut sugar or a few drops lemon stevia (optional)

Blueberry Protein Chocolate Shake

This is my husband's favorite smoothie. It gets him through his daily run and a solid morning of work. As he says, he can go all day on this one. He's taught several of his guy friends how to make it—that's how deep his healthy addiction goes. The plant-based protein from hemp and chia seeds is easily absorbed by your body. The added maca root powder gives an extra energy boost. The cacao powder is high in antioxidants and adds a nice hint of chocolate. Blueberries add phytonutrients and the banana adds potassium and sweetness.

Preparation: Combine all ingredients in a blender and process at high speed until smooth. Makes 1 serving.

Ingredients:

1 scoop hemp protein powder
1 tbsp maca powder
1 tbsp chia seeds
1 tsp raw cacao powder
1 c organic almond milk or non-dairy milk
1 banana, frozen
1/2 c frozen blueberries
1 tsp vanilla extract
pinch cinnamon (optional)
1 tsp raw unsweetened coconut

Ingredients:

2 c almond milk or coco-
nut milk

3 tbsp liquid coconut sugar, or
15 drops liquid vanilla stevia, or 3 tbsp maple syrup

1/2 c whole chia seeds

1 tsp vanilla extract

pinch sea salt

1 tsp raw cacao powder

1 c berries (raspberries,
blackberries, or blueber-
ries), plus extra for topping

1/2 c nuts or seeds for
topping

1 tsp ground cinnamon for
topping

Chia Seed Pudding with Summer Berries

I love this chia seed pudding. It's easy to make, it tastes great, and it's a healthy treat. My son is crazy for it and enjoys it often as breakfast. He takes it along and eats it on the drive to school.

Preparation: In a 1-quart mason jar or other container with a tight-fitting lid, combine the almond milk or coconut milk and sweetener of your choice. Shake well to combine. Add the chia seeds, vanilla extract, sea salt, cacao, and berries. Shake well to combine all ingredients. Refrigerate for at least 4 hours or overnight. When the pudding thickens, it's ready. To serve, spoon the pudding into small bowls. Top with additional berries and seeds or nuts; sprinkle with the cinnamon. Makes 4 servings.

Ingredients:

2 small limes or 1 large
lime including peel,
organic only

1 avocado, peeled and
sliced

1 c ice cubes or crushed ice

1 packet (1 g) stevia

Raw and Healthy Lime Sherbet

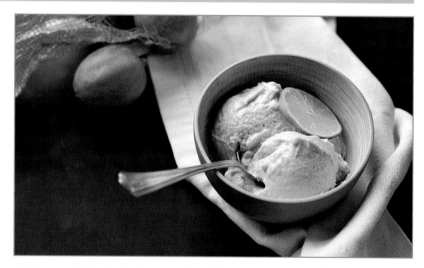

This sherbet is inspired by my friend Theresa, a local raw foodie and super-healthy, ageless beauty. She whipped this up for me at her house on a hot summer afternoon. I couldn't wait to get home to my Vitamix to put my own spin on it. Here's my variation, inspired by Theresa. It's incredibly delicious, refreshing, good for you, and guilt-free.

Preparation: Combine all the ingredients in a juicer or high-speed blender. Process on high until the ice is blended in. Serve immediately. Makes 1 serving.

Heirloom Tomato Salad

Executive Chef Jonathan Senigen of Eliza-beth's Gone Raw restaurant in Washington, DC, created this recipe. The restaurant is one of my favorites. Founder Elizabeth Petty is an inspiration and a leader in the local raw food and vegan community. This tomato salad is the perfect way to use the abundant fresh toma-toes of summer. The hemp dressing is delicious; store the extra in a glass container in your refrigerator.

Ingredients:

Salad:
3 large, fresh tomatoes, seeded and cut into bite-sized pieces
1 tbsp walnut oil
sea salt to taste
white pepper to taste
3 tbsp fresh lemon juice
2 fennel bulbs, cored and thinly sliced
1 tsp fresh marjoram leaves

Vinaigrette:
1 c hemp seeds
4 c water
1 tbsp dry mustard
1/2 shallot
1½ c soaked cashews (soak overnight in the refrigerator in water to cover)
sea salt to taste
white pepper to taste

Preparation: In a large bowl, toss the tomato pieces with the walnut oil, sea salt and white pepper to taste, and half the lemon juice. In a separate bowl, combine the fen-nel slices with the remaining lemon juice, marjoram leaves, and sea salt and white pepper to taste. To make the dressing, drain the cashews. Combine the cashews, hemp seeds, water, mustard, and shallot in a blender. Process until smooth. Season to taste with sea salt and white pepper. To serve the salad, place half of the vinaigrette into the bottom of each of four serving bowls. Arrange 1/4 of the tomato mixture in each bowl and top each with 1/4 of the fennel mixture. Makes 4 servings.

Chard and Sheep Cheese

I invented this recipe years ago out of desperation when the community-supported agriculture farm I belonged to had a big year for chard. There were only so many green smoothies I could make with the huge pile of chard leaves that arrived each week. This dish was a hit with my family—finally, they enjoyed chard as much as I do. If no chard is available, try making this recipes with fresh spinach instead.

Ingredients:

1½ lbs chard
sea salt to taste
cayenne pepper to taste
2 tbsp extra-virgin olive oil
1/2 c shredded raw sheep cheese

Preparation: Preheat oven to 450°F. Bring a large pot of water to a boil. Trim the chard and remove tough stems. Cut the leaves into 2-inch strips. Blanch the chard in the boiling water for 2 to 3 minutes. Drain in a colander and press gently to remove excess water. Grease a 9-inch baking dish with 1 tsp of the olive oil. Place the chard in the dish and season to taste with sea salt and cayenne pepper. Drizzle with the remaining olive oil and toss to coat the leaves. Sprinkle the cheese over the top and bake for 10 minutes, or until the cheese is lightly browned. Makes 4 servings.

Ingredients:

Salad:

1 medium zucchini, peeled into ribbons with a vegetable peeler

1 medium summer squash, peeled into ribbons with a vegetable peeler

1 large carrot, peeled into ribbons with a vegetable peeler

4 oz organic baby romaine lettuce

Fresh marinara sauce:

5 large, fresh tomatoes, seeded and cut into chunks

5 unsulfured sun-dried tomatoes, soaked in 1 c water for 10 minutes and drained

1 tbsp fresh oregano

1/4 c loosely packed fresh basil leaves

1 tbsp fresh rosemary

1 heaping tbsp chopped fresh ginger

2 garlic cloves

2 tbsp cold-pressed olive oil

1 tsp soy sauce or tamari

1 tsp sea salt

stevia to taste

Squash Pasta with Raw Tomato Sauce

This recipe is courtesy of Natalia Rose, best-selling author of *The Raw Food Detox Diet* and *Forever Beautiful: The Age-Defying Detox Plan*. She calls this dish "the amazing marinara cell-cleanse" because it's so full of healthy antioxidants. Natalia's recipe calls for soy sauce or tamari; if you want to avoid soy, use an equal amount of coconut aminos (a soy-free substitute for soy sauce made from coconuts—look for it in the health food store).

Preparation: Combine the zucchini, summer squash, carrot, and romaine in a large serving bowl. Toss gently to combine. Combine the fresh tomatoes, sun-dried tomatoes, oregano, basil, rosemary, ginger, garlic, olive oil, soy sauce or tamari, sea salt, and stevia in a blender or food processor. Process on high until smooth. Pour the fresh marinara sauce over the vegetables in the bowl. Toss well to coat vegetables. Serve immediately. Makes 2 servings.

Ingredients:

1¼ lbs ground turkey

1 c mushroom caps, coarsely chopped

3 shallots, coarsely chopped

1/2 c coarsely chopped kale

1 tsp tamari sauce

sea salt to taste

cayenne pepper to taste

1/2 tsp powdered ginger

1 tsp coconut oil

Nutritional Style Turkey Burgers

My son used to attend a polo camp when he was little. The Argentine owners and players loved to cook burgers for the kids. On my advice, they added slivers of kale to the burgers to boost their nutrients. That's a good start, but I take it a step further. I make my burgers from ground turkey with kale and add mushrooms and onions for a tender, moist burger. If you want to avoid soy, substitute coconut aminos for the tamari. Serve on gluten-free buns along with sweet potato fries (see recipe on page 188) and a green salad.

Preparation: Put the ground turkey in a large mixing bowl and add the mushrooms, shallots, kale, tamari, sea salt, cayenne pepper, and ginger. Gently mix the ingredients until well blended. Divide the turkey mixture into 4 balls, then press the balls into patties. Put the patties on a plate, cover, and refrigerate until firm, about 30 minutes. To cook, heat the coconut oil in a large sauté pan until it melts. Add the burgers and cook for 5 to 7 minutes. Turn and cook for another 5 minutes. Makes 4 servings.

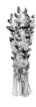

Yellow Squash Fettuccini with Creamy Pine Nut Alfredo

I once had the honor of spending an evening in the kitchen of the Pure Food and Wine restaurant in New York City, observing, helping, and trying to stay out of the way of chef Sarma Melngailis as she created her magic raw dishes. She does the same at her other New York restaurant, One Lucky Duck Take-Away. If you can't dine with Sarma, you can read her wonderful cookbook, *Living Raw Food*. Sarma contributed this recipe—it's a great way to share the benefits of raw food with the uninitiated. This dish is remarkable: a creamy, rich, and satisfying pasta dish without the flour and gluten of regular pasta or the dairy, cheese, and butter of a traditional Alfredo sauce.

Preparation: To make the Alfredo sauce, place the pine nuts in a bowl and add enough water to cover. Let sit for an hour or more to plump the nuts. Drain the pine nuts and put them in the blender along with the olive oil, lemon juice, nutritional yeast, and sea salt. Blend until smooth. If the sauce is too thick, stir in a bit of water to thin it. To make the squash fettuccini, trim the squash. Julienne them on a mandolin, or use a vegetable peeler to make them into ribbons, or use a spiral slicer to cut them into broad slices. Place the squash fettuccini into a colander and toss with 1/2 tsp sea salt. Let stand for at least 30 minutes to soften and allow a bit of the liquid to drain off. In a small bowl, toss the chopped pine nuts with the oil and the remaining sea salt. Place enough squash fettuccini for two servings in a medium bowl. Add enough of the Alfredo sauce to generously coat the squash fettuccini. Add the capers and half the basil; season to taste with black pepper. Toss gently. To serve, divide the squash fettuccini between two shallow bowls, making tall piles. Drizzle more of the sauce on the squash, sprinkle with the chopped pine nuts, and garnish with the remaining basil leaves. Makes 2 servings.

Ingredients:

Alfredo sauce:
1 ½ c raw pine nuts
3 tbsp olive oil
3 tbsp fresh lemon juice
1 tbsp nutritional yeast
1/2 tsp sea salt

Squash fettuccini:
2 to 3 medium yellow summer squash
1 tsp sea salt
1/4 c raw pine nuts, coarsely chopped
1/2 tsp walnut oil or olive oil
1/4 c small capers
1/2 c lemon or regular basil leaves
black pepper to taste

Avocado and Cucumber Soup

Although I love to eat seasonally, I enjoy this creamy soup year-round. It's easy to make and very satisfying. This can be a delicious first course or a tasty lunch or dinner, served with a side salad. My Modern Vegan friends adore this recipe because it's raw, yet I can serve it at a dinner party to a roomful of people with various Nutritional Styles.

Preparation: Place the avocado, cucumber, green onions, garlic, lemon juice, and water in a blender. Process until smooth; add a bit more water if you prefer a thinner soup. Add sea salt and cayenne pepper to taste. Chill the soup in the refrigerator for at least 1 hour. Garnish the serving bowls with sprigs of cilantro. Makes 2 servings.

Ingredients:

2 ripe avocados, peeled and seeded
1/2 large cucumber, peeled and thickly sliced
5 green onions (bottoms only), chopped
1 garlic clove
3 tbsp lemon juice
1 c water
sea salt to taste
cayenne pepper to taste (optional)
cilantro sprigs

Ingredients:

2 to 3 large sweet
   potatoes
1 tbsp olive oil
sea salt to taste
ground cinnamon to taste
   (optional)
maple syrup for dipping
   (optional)

Sweet Potato Fries

Did you know that sweet root vegetables like carrots, sweet potatoes, and butternut squash are not only high in vitamin A and beta carotene (think gorgeous skin!) but also a great way to keep sugar cravings at bay? They're all high in natural sugars—the good kind that doesn't spike your blood glucose—and that keeps you from wanting processed sweets such as cookies and candy later on. I often recommend increasing root vegetables to my clients who suffer from sugar cravings. It really works. Here's an easy recipe for my favorite way to enjoy a delicious sweet potato. This recipe works just as well for white potatoes or carrots.

Preparation: Preheat oven to 350°F. Peel the sweet potatoes and slice them into long strips about 1/4 inch thick. Place the olive oil in a large mixing bowl. Add the sweet potato strips and toss to coat. Sprinkle with sea salt. For an even sweeter taste, sprinkle with ground cinnamon. Spread the fries evenly on a baking sheet. Bake until golden brown, about 25 minutes. Turn once, carefully, after 15 minutes. Serve with maple syrup for dipping. Makes 2 servings.

Ingredients:

Truffles:
1/2 c coconut oil, warmed
   gently in a saucepan to
   soften
3/4 c coconut nectar
   (liquid coconut sugar)
2 tsp vanilla extract
8 drops vanilla stevia
1/4 tsp sea salt
1 c dried shredded coconut
2¼ c raw cocoa powder,
   sifted

Toppings:
1/4 c raw shredded coconut
1/4 c raw cocoa nibs
1/4 c hemp seeds
1/4 c raw cocoa powder

Superfood Cacao Truffles

Sometimes I make these truffles just to keep on hand as an easy and healthy treat; one rich bite and my cravings for sweets seem to disappear. I've taken them to TV appearances, speaking engagements, my friends' homes, and elsewhere—everyone loves them. If I'm feeling fancy, I double the recipe and make the full assortment of superfood toppings, then arrange the truffles on a beautiful tray. They make a gorgeous impression. Modern Vegans enjoy these truffles because they have a rich, chocolatey taste without any butter or cream.

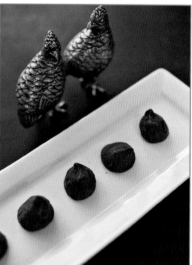

Preparation: Combine warmed coconut oil, coconut nectar, vanilla extract, and salt in a blender. Blend briefly at high speed until mixed. Add 1/2 c shredded coconut and blend until smooth; add the remaining 1/2 c and blend again until smooth. Transfer the mixture to a large mixing bowl and stir in 2 c of the cocoa powder until combined. Cover the bowl and refrigerate for 15 minutes or until the mixture is firm. In the meantime, place the different toppings into shallow bowls. To make the truffles, use your palms to roll heaping tablespoons of the mixture into balls. Roll the truffles in the toppings to coat. Store the truffles in the refrigerator or freezer. Makes about 35 truffles.

Sweet Pea and Avocado Guacamole

One of my favorite spas, Rancho la Puerta near San Diego, has been making a version of this guacamole for years, adding various vegetables to traditional guacamole to boost the nutrients. I like to make this in the spring with fresh peas, but you can substitute edamame, cooked broccoli, or even cooked asparagus.

Preparation: Process the peas in a blender or food processor until smooth. Place the peas into a large mixing bowl. Mash the avocado in a small bowl and add it to the mixing bowl. Add the lime juice, onion, jalapeño pepper, cilantro, and garlic. Blend well with a spoon. Season to taste with sea salt and cayenne pepper. Makes about 2 cups.

Ingredients:

1 c fresh peas
1 medium avocado, peeled and pitted
2 tbsp fresh lime juice or to taste
1/2 red or sweet onion, finely diced
1 jalapeño pepper, seeded and finely chopped
1/4 c fresh cilantro, coarsely chopped
1 garlic clove, finely chopped
sea salt to taste
cayenne pepper to taste

Vegetable Frittata

When I was a kid, my Italian dad made a big frittata every year on Easter Sunday. He could make frittatas better than anyone, and we anticipated it as much as our Easter baskets full of candy. (Well, maybe not that much.) Although Dad's frittata often included Italian pepperoni, he always added lots of greens, too. Spinach or parsley were his favorites—they still are. Here's my healthier version, which adds more greens and skips the pepperoni.

Preparation: Preheat oven to 350°F. In an ovenproof skillet or sauté pan, heat the olive oil and add the onion. Cook, stirring often, until the onion is softened. Add the kale, the other vegetables of your choice, and the red pepper. Cook, stirring often, until the vegetables are tender. In a mixing bowl, whisk together the eggs, herbes de Provence, sea salte, and cayenne or black pepper. Pour the mixture over the vegetables in the pan and stir gently to blend. Sprinkle with the cheese if you're using it. Bake for 25 minutes, or until the eggs puff up and the top is lightly browned. To serve, slice the frittata in the pan as if it were a pie. Alternatively, let the pan cool slightly, then place a sturdy serving plate over it. Flip the pan and plate over to move the frittata onto the plate for slicing. Makes 6 servings.

Ingredients:

1 tbsp extra-virgin olive oil
1/2 sweet onion, peeled and thinly sliced
2 c kale leaves, stems removed and chopped into thin slivers
2 c vegetables of your choice, such as cauliflower, zucchini, or broccoli, cut into small pieces
1 red pepper, seeded and cut into 1/2 inch pieces
12 organic, pasture-raised eggs
2 tbsp herbes de Provence (a mixture of garlic, lavender, lemon peel, oregano, sea salt, and other aromatic herbs)
sea salt to taste
cayenne pepper or black pepper to taste
3 oz goat cheese or grated sheep cheese (optional)

Fall Recipes

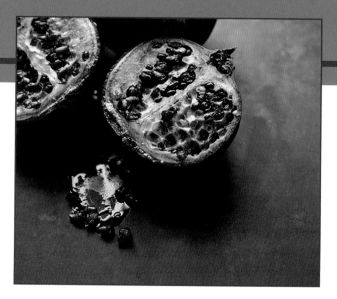

You know that time of year when salads begin to feel chilly to your system? As fall arrives, warm up your digestion with a harvest of warming, stick-to-your-ribs foods, especially if they're fresh and local. Autumn bounty is colorful and rich in flavor. It's the ideal time to boost your nutritional profile with an array of phytonutrients and sweet and savory flavors from pumpkins, butternut squash, carrots, apples, and pomegranates.

Ingredients:

1 c fresh or frozen pomegranate seeds
1 frozen banana
2 medjool dates, pitted
2 c hemp milk or other non-dairy milk
1 scoop hemp protein
1 tbsp ground flaxseed
1 tbsp chia seeds
dash cayenne pepper

Sweet Pomegranate Smoothie

Pomegranate seeds are a bit messy to prepare (see page 137 for how to do this). Fortunately, the health food store near my home now sells fresh pomegranate seeds (frozen seeds are also available). Call me lazy, but that has led me to make this pretty pink smoothie much more often in the fall, when pomegranates are abundant. Using medjool dates as the sweetener adds a depth of flavor that's almost candy like.

Preparation: Combine the pomegranate seeds, banana, dates, hemp milk, hemp protein, flaxseed, chia seeds, and cayenne pepper in a blender. Process at high speed until smooth. Makes 2 servings.

Ingredients:

4 fresh apples (such as Honey Crisp, Fuji, Rome, or for a tart taste, Granny Smith)
Nutmeg, cinnamon, or pumpkin pie spice

Easy Baked Apple Rings

I raised my son on apples cut into cubes and sprinkled with cinnamon. In fact, I used to send him to school with "apple pie apples" every single day. It was a great way to disguise the browning of the cut apples (a natural and safe enzymatic reaction) and encourage him to eat them. He finally figured out what I was doing at about age 12, but he still asks for them. Some days, I bake apples in rings and the entire house smells like apple pie.

Preparation: Preheat the oven to 200°F. Peel and core the apples, then slice them into thin rings. Line a baking sheet with parchment paper. Arrange the apple rings on the sheet and sprinkle generously with the spices of your choice. Bake for 30 minutes. Using a spatula, gently turn the apple rings. Sprinkle again with the spices and bake for 30 more minutes. Store any leftovers in the refrigerator. Makes 4 servings.

Pantry Granola

Granola is good for you, but the commercial versions, even the so-called healthy ones, are loaded with added sugar and unhealthy fats. My husband loves granola, especially the kind with oats. My son, well, he's a kid, so he loves any kind of cereal. To make sure they're getting a healthy version of their favorite breakfast food, I make my own granola. I like to add dried fruit to the mix. Any dried fruit, alone or in combination, will work. Try goji berries, cherries, cranberries, raisins, or golden berries. I try to keep a stock in my pantry, but it never lasts long. Fortunately, this recipe is quick and easy to make.

Preparation: Preheat oven to 350°F. In a very large mixing bowl, combine the oats, maple sugar, honey or maple syrup, coconut flakes, vanilla, and flaxseed. Gently heat 3/4 c coconut oil in a small saucepan until it is just liquefied and add it to the mixture. Mix well to combine the ingredients and coat them with the coconut oil. Grease two cookie sheets with the remaining 1 tbsp coconut oil. Spread the granola mixture evenly on the cookie sheets. Bake for 30 minutes, stirring with a spatula a few times to brown the granola evenly. Remove from the oven and let cool for a few minutes. Stir in the dried fruit, sea salt, and crushed nuts or seeds if using them. Let cool completely and store in an air-tight container in the refrigerator. Makes 8 cups.

Ingredients:

4 c gluten-free organic raw oats
3/4 c plus 1 tbsp coconut oil
1/2 c maple sugar
1/2 c raw honey or pure maple syrup
2 c unsweetened coconut flakes
1 tbsp vanilla extract
1/2 cup flaxseed
1 c dried fruit
1 c crushed nuts or seeds (optional)
sea salt to taste

"Cheesy" Kale Chips

These chips, perfect for Flexible Vegetarians and Modern Vegans, are so good that in my house they never make it from the stove to the pantry. My guys eat them straight from the baking trays while standing in the kitchen. This is a great way to use the kale that's still abundant in the early autumn.

Preparation: Preheat oven to 400°F. Trim tough stems from the kale and tear the leaves into 2-inch pieces. In a large mixing bowl, toss the kale in the olive oil, making sure each piece is lightly coated. Spread the kale pieces in one layer on baking sheets and sprinkle them with sea salt and the nutritional yeast. Bake, stirring gently a few times, until the kale pieces are light brown and crisp, about 20 minutes. Be careful not to burn. To make a raw version of the chips, prepare the kale as for baking and put the pieces in a dehydrator set at 115°F. Dehydrate until the kale is very crispy, about 6 to 8 hours. Store the chips in an airtight container in the pantry. Makes about 6 cups.

Ingredients:

1 big bunch kale
2 tbsp extra-virgin olive oil
sea salt to taste
3 tbsp nutritional yeast

Banana Buttercup Smoothie with Kale

Puree Artisan Juice Bar is a favorite foodie spot in DC. I'm there so often that I keep a special container in my kitchen to recycle their adorable glass juice bottles. They press their fresh, organic juices daily—and deliver them to my door, too. This smoothie, created by proprietor Amy Waldman, is my son's favorite, but please don't tell him about the kale.

Preparation: Combine the banana, almond milk, cacao nibs, kale, almond butter, and ground cinnamon in a blender. Process at high speed until smooth. Makes 1 serving.

Ingredients:

1 frozen banana
9 oz almond milk
1/2 oz cacao nibs, or more for taste and texture
1 c kale leaves
2 tbsp almond butter
ground cinnamon to taste

Ingredients:

1 tbsp olive oil
1 c diced sweet onion
1 head cauliflower, roughly
    chopped
2 c vegetable broth
1 c coconut milk
sea salt to taste
rosemary sprig or nutmeg
    to taste

Holli's Famous Creamy Cauliflower Soup

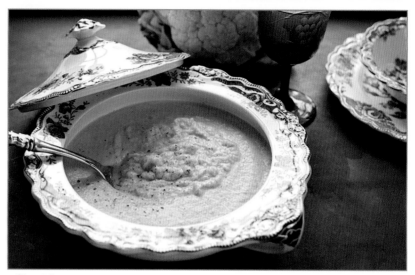

Cauliflower soup is very quick and easy to make. The coconut milk gives this soup a creamy texture that's ideal for Flexible Vegetarians and Modern Vegans who want to avoid dairy products. The soup makes a wonderful lunch or light supper. I've given the recipe to many clients and posted it on my blog; it's beloved by everyone who tries it. I use organic coconut milk, which can be hard to find. If it's not available, make your own using raw coconut flakes—here's my recipe.

Preparation: Heat the olive oil in a pot and add the diced onion. Sauté until the onion is golden around the edges. Add the cauliflower and the broth to the pot. The broth should just cover the cauliflower. Simmer over low heat until the cauliflower is very tender. Transfer the mixture, in batches if necessary, to a blender or food processor and process until smooth and creamy. Return the mixture to the pot and add the coconut milk and sea salt. Cook until the soup is hot. Serve immediately, garnished with a rosemary sprig or a dash of nutmeg. Makes 4 servings.

Ingredients:

4 c filtered water
2 c raw, unsweetened,
    organic shredded or
    flaked coconut
1 tsp vanilla extract
    (optional)

DIY Coconut Milk

This non-dairy milk is super simple. I sometimes don't bother to strain it if I plan to use it for smoothies. Store coconut milk in a glass container in the refrigerator. Stir well before using. It will keep well for a week.

Preparation: Put the water, coconut, and vanilla extract in a blender. Blend on high for 1 to 2 minutes. Strain the mixture using a nut-milk bag or cheesecloth bag.

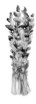

Autumn Harvest Soup

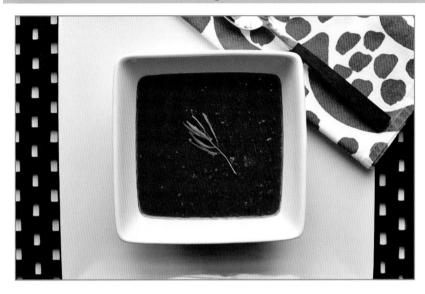

Ingredients:

2 large red peppers, seeded and diced

4 carrots, sliced

2 fresh tomatoes, seeded and diced

2 c plain coconut milk or almond milk

1/2 c raw cashews

1 small hot pepper, seeded and finely diced

1 garlic clove

1 tbsp lemon juice

sea salt to taste

1 avocado, peeled and thinly sliced

I'm crazy for this easy harvest soup, made with the freshest ingredients straight from your garden or the farmers' market. Nutritionally, it's all here: vitamin C for your immune system from the red peppers, beta carotene for beautiful skin from the carrots, and heart-healthy lycopene from the tomatoes. Add in some raw cashews for a protein boost and you have the perfect meal.

Preparation: Combine the peppers, carrots, tomatoes, coconut milk, cashews, hot pepper, garlic clove, and lemon juice in a blender or food processor. Season to taste with sea salt. Process until the mixture is smooth. Serve gently warmed or cold, garnished with the avocado slices. Makes 2 servings.

Butternut Squash and Apple Soup

Ingredients:

1 large (2 to 3 pounds) butternut squash, peeled and seeded

2 tbsp extra-virgin olive oil

1 medium onion, chopped

1 apple, peeled and chopped

6 c vegetable stock

nutmeg to taste

cinnamon to taste

sea salt to taste

black pepper to taste (optional)

This seasonal soup is warming and aromatic; it's rich in beta carotene and fiber from the butternut squash, and the boost of vitamin C from the apples helps strengthen your immunity. It's just what you need this fall to keep you and your family healthy. My son loves this soup because it's a little bit sweet, but then again, he loves anything with apples in it.

Preparation: Cut the squash into 1-inch chunks. In a large pot, heat the olive oil and add the onion. Cook until the onion is translucent, about 8 minutes. Add the squash, apple, and stock. Bring to a simmer and cook until the squash is tender, about 15 to 20 minutes. Remove the squash chunks with a slotted spoon and place them in a blender. Puree (or use your hand-held or immersion blender in the pot). Return blended squash to pot. Stir well and season to taste with nutmeg, cinnamon, salt, and black pepper. Makes 4 servings.

Ingredients:

4 medium zucchini, halved
  lengthwise and thinly sliced
4 medium yellow summer
  squash, halved length-
  wise and thinly sliced
4 shallots, thinly sliced
4 tbsp extra-virgin olive oil
2 tsp fresh thyme leaves
12 thin lemon slices
8 tsp lemon juice
sea salt to taste
cayenne pepper to taste
4 skinless salmon fillets (4
  to 5 oz each)

Wild Salmon and Zucchini in Parchment

I love to serve this dish to Healthy Omnivores and Flexible Vegetarians. There's something about opening the parchment wrap that makes guests feel like you're giving them a gift, which of course you are. Zucchini and summer squash are still plentiful in the early days of autumn; they add a light but satisfying accompaniment to the wild salmon. I serve this dish with a large salad in a delicate apple cider and mustard vinaigrette (see recipe on this page).

Preparation: Preheat oven to 350°F. For each fillet, fold a large piece of parchment paper (about 15 by 16 inches) in half to crease it; open, and lay it flat. On one side of the crease pile 1/4 of the squash and zucchini, top with 1/4 of the shallots, drizzle with 2 tbsp olive oil, and sprinkle with sea salt and cayenne pepper. Place a fillet on top, skin-side down, drizzle with 2 tsp lemon juice, and season with additional sea salt and cayenne pepper. Fold the parchment over the salmon, make small overlapping folds to seal the open sides, and create a half-moon-shaped packet. Repeat for the other 3 pieces. Place the parchments on a baking sheet with a rim. Bake for 15 minutes. To serve, place the parchment packages on individual serving dishes and slice open at the table to reveal the fish and vegetables. Makes 4 servings.

Ingredients:

Salad:
1 lb brussels sprouts
1 c roughly chopped raw
  pecans
1/2 c dried cranberries
1/3 c crumbled raw goat
  cheese
Dressing:
6 tbsp extra-virgin olive oil
2 tbsp apple cider vinegar
2 tsp Dijon mustard
sea salt to taste
cayenne pepper to taste

Cleansing Brussels Sprouts Salad with Pecans, Cranberries, and Goat Cheese

Brussels sprouts are deliciously high in vitamin C and fiber, along with live enzymes and a rich array of phytonutrients. This salad is a favorite combination of crunchy, sweet, and savory flavors. It's best in the late fall, when the brussels sprouts are being harvested and are at their most flavorful.

Preparation: Trim the brussels sprouts. Slice them into thin ribbons. Put the slices into a large mixing bowl. Add the pecans, dried cranberries, and goat cheese to the bowl and toss lightly to mix. In a small mixing bowl, whisk together the olive oil, cider vinegar, Dijon mustard, sea salt, and cayenne pepper. Pour the dressing over the brussels sprouts mixture and toss until all the ingredients are well coated. Serve immediately. Makes 4 servings.

Ingredients:

1/2 c extra-virgin olive oil
1/2 c organic apple cider
  vinegar
1/4 tsp sea salt
1/2 tsp organic Dijon
  mustard
1 garlic clove
1/4 c coconut syrup

Apple Cider and Mustard Vinaigrette

This piquant salad dressing contains apple cider vinegar, a healthy choice for your digestion. Use the best organic extra-virgin olive oil you can afford. The coconut syrup rounds out the flavor. This dressing keeps well in the fridge for several days.

Preparation: Combine the olive oil, apple cider vinegar, sea salt, mustard, garlic cloves, and coconut syrup in a blender. Process on high until smooth. Makes 1 cup

Winter Recipes

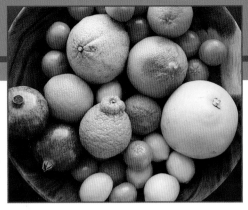

Relax, rest, and stay warm this winter by doing what you're programmed to do: sleep more and enjoy heartier foods that warm you from the inside out. Winter's harvest is rooted deep in the earth. Now's the season for root vegetables. It's time to use them in soups and stews that make for friendly dinners on cold, snowy, or damp days. Don't forget your dark leafy greens and citrus fruits now, to help you keep your nutrition and immunity strong.

Skinny Green Smoothie

Ingredients:

I love grapefruit and I often crave it in the winter months, when local produce is scarce. That tells me that I'm needing the vitamin C and fresh flavor grapefruit offers. Fortunately, winter is the season for citrus fruit. A word of warning: A surprisingly long list of prescription drugs have bad interactions with grapefruit juice. If you take any prescription medications, check with your doctor before making this smoothie part of your life. You could substitute two peeled oranges for the grapefruit if you like.

Preparation: Combine the romaine lettuce, cucumber, kale, grapefruit, and water in a blender. Process on high until the mixture is smooth. Store the extra in a glass container in the refrigerator; use it the same day. Makes 1 quart.

- 1 head romaine lettuce
- 1 large cucumber
- 4 kale leaves
- 1 grapefruit, peeled
- 16 to 20 oz pure water

Healing Tea with Turmeric and Ginger

Ingredients:

Turmeric, the spice that gives curry powder its yellow color, has powerful anti-inflammatory properties. Ginger has both anti-inflammatory and antibiotic properties. Together they make a potent healing combination. Try it when you're down with a winter cold—the zingy flavor will help you feel better.

Preparation: Heat the water in a small saucepan until it is nearly boiling. Add the ginger and turmeric. Lower the heat and simmer for 10 minutes. Strain the liquid into a mug and stir in the honey and lemon juice. Drink while still hot. Makes 2 servings.

- 2 cups water
- 1/2 tsp grated fresh ginger
- 1/2 tsp turmeric
- 1 tbsp raw, local honey
- 1 tbsp fresh lemon juice

Ingredients:

1/2 avocado, peeled and sliced

2 c almond milk

1 tbsp maca powder

1 tbsp hemp seeds

1 tbsp raw cacao

3 medjool dates, pitted

10 drops liquid vanilla stevia

dash ground cinnamon

Chocolate and Avocado Smoothie

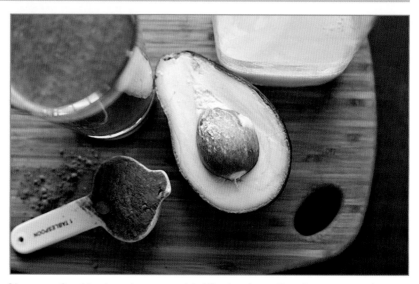

I'm crazy for this chocolate smoothie. The key ingredient is maca powder, a root that is known to increase energy and virility, if that's your thing. (I explain more about maca powder in the list of superfoods on page 175.) I find maca gives me a powerful boost on days when I need to be calm but brave, such as when I have to stand in front of a TV camera or watch my son's tennis match.

Preparation: Combine the avocado, almond milk, maca powder, hemp seeds, cacao, dates, stevia, and cinnamon in a blender. Process at high speed until smooth. Store the extra in a glass container in the refrigerator; use it the same day. Makes 2 servings.

Ingredients:

1 tbsp coconut oil

15 oz cooked black beans

2 large, ripe bananas

1/3 c coconut sugar

1/4 c raw cacao powder

1 tbsp raw cacao nibs

1 tsp vanilla extract

1 tbsp ground cinnamon

3 tbsp local honey

1/4 tsp sea salt

1/4 c instant rolled oats

1/4 c crushed walnuts (optional)

Black Bean Brownies

One of my clients, a dedicated Flexible Vegetarian, gave me her recipe for black bean brownies because I didn't believe her when she told me how everybody loved them. I stand corrected. Even my son and his friends admit that they're delicious, albeit a bit weird. I probably shouldn't have shared the main ingredient with them, but they devour them anyway. They go fast—make lots.

Preparation: Preheat oven to 350°F. Grease a 9-inch baking pan with the coconut oil. Combine the black beans, bananas, coconut sugar, cacao powder, cacao nibs, vanilla, cinnamon, honey, and sea salt in a food processor or blender. Process until smooth. Put the mixture into a mixing bowl and gently stir in the oats. Press the mixture evenly into the pan and sprinkle the top with crushed walnuts, if using them. Bake for 30 minutes, or until browned on top.

Easy Green Bars

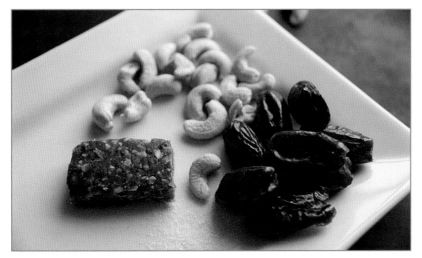

Ingredients:

2 c raw cashews
2 c medjool dates, pitted
4 tsp organic green pow-
    der, such as spirulina,
    chlorella, or wheatgrass
2 tbsp lemon juice
1 tbsp lemon zest

I add veggies and greens to whatever I can, and that includes snacks and treats. These easy green snack bars are a standby in my house. In this recipe, I give the basic version using an organic green powder (see my list of superfoods on page 174 for more information). Once you get the idea, get creative with added healthy ingredients, such as goji berries, golden berries, or raisins. I think the green color is fun, but if you get pushback from your family, just call them alien bars. They'll eat them anyway, they're that good.

Preparation: Process the cashews in a food processor until they are finely ground (stop processing before the nuts turn to butter). Add the dates, green powder, and lemon juice and process until the mixture forms a large ball. Add the lemon zest and process until just blended. Line an 8 x 12 baking dish with wax paper or parchment paper. Press the bar mixture firmly and evenly into the dish. Refrigerate for 30 minutes to 1 hour, or until the bars are firm. Cut into bars or squares. Store in the fridge in a glass container. The bars freeze well. Makes 8 servings.

Chocolate and Banana Quinoa Cereal

Ingredients:

My son was iffy on quinoa until I began adding chocolate and banana to it. Now this is one of his favorite breakfasts. You can top this with additional coconut milk or any non-dairy milk of your choice for a creamier texture.

Preparation: Combine the almond, hemp, or coconut milk with the water in a saucepan. Bring to a boil and stir in the quinoa and sea salt. Reduce the heat to low, cover, and simmer 8 to 10 minutes, or until the liquid is absorbed. Stir occasionally. Put the cooked quinoa into a mixing bowl. Add the banana slices (save a few for garnish), the coconut sugar, cacao powder, vanilla, and cinnamon. Stir well, mashing in the banana. Divide between 2 individual serving bowls and garnish with banana slices. Makes 2 servings.

1 c almond, hemp, or
    coconut milk
1/2 c water
1/2 c raw quinoa
sea salt to taste
1 banana, sliced
2 tsp coconut sugar
2 tsp raw cacao powder
1/2 tsp vanilla extract
dash ground cinnamon

Ingredients:

Cleansing Salad

Salad:

1 head broccoli, trimmed and broken into florets

1 head cauliflower, trimmed and broken into florets

2 large carrots

1/2 c sunflower seeds or slivered almonds

1 c dried berries of your choice, such as cranberries or golden berries

1/2 c dried blueberries

1/2 c finely chopped fresh parsley

Dressing:

6 tbsp lemon juice

1 tbsp extra-virgin olive oil

sea salt to taste

cayenne pepper to taste

raw, local honey to taste (optional)

This hearty salad is a great way to enjoy raw cruciferous vegetables and their disease-fighting properties. Broccoli, cauliflower, and carrots are good winter choices at the market. This salad keeps well for several days in the fridge. In fact, it gets better as the flavors meld. If you're a Healthy Omnivore, you can add pieces of chicken breast, turkey, or any other cooked meat to the salad—a great way to use up leftovers.

Preparation: Finely chop the broccoli and cauliflower florets in a food processor or by hand. Shred the carrots in a food processor or by hand with a grater. Put the broccoli, cauliflower, and carrots into a large mixing bowl. Add the sunflower seeds, golden berries, parsley, and blueberries. In a small bowl, whisk together the lemon juice, olive oil, sea salt, and cayenne pepper. Drizzle in honey to taste if you wish. Pour the dressing over the vegetables and toss gently to mix. Let stand for at least 1 hour to let the flavors meld. Makes 10 servings.

Ingredients:

Baked Cod with Olive and Caper Pesto

1 c pitted Kalamata olives

1/4 c capers, drained

1 tbsp lemon zest

3 tbsp lemon juice

1 c roughly chopped fresh parsley

2 garlic cloves

1/2 c raw walnuts

1/4 c extra-virgin olive oil

4 4- to 6-oz cod fillets

Dr. Mark Hyman, author of *The Blood Sugar Solution* and six other bestselling books, is an internationally recognized leader, speaker, educator, and advocate in the field of functional medicine. He's the founder and medical director of the UltraWellness Center, chairman of the board of the Institute for Functional Medicine, medical editor of *The Huffington Post,* and a regular guest on television discussing current health issues. I'm delighted to have this recipe from him! Healthy Omnivores and Flexible Vegetarians can substitute any firm white fish for the cod.

Preparation: Preheat oven to 350°F. In a food processor, combine the olives, capers, lemon zest, lemon juice, parsley, garlic, and walnuts. Process for 20 seconds. Drizzle in the olive oil while the motor is running; pulse to combine. Spread about 1 tbsp of the olive and caper pesto onto each fish fillet. Place the fish in a greased ovenproof dish. Bake for 20 minutes. Makes 4 servings.

Soba Noodles with Creamy Nut Sauce

This is a quick standby dinner in my house. It's also a treat for me, both because it tastes great and is very easy to prepare. I almost always have all the ingredients on hand. The sauce takes just a few minutes to blend. If you have leftover sauce (or care to double the recipe, as I often do), save it for the next day to dress your salad, or warm it and serve over steamed vegetables. Soba noodles are Japanese noodles made from buckwheat; they should be avoided if you are gluten intolerant. If you're OK with gluten and don't have soba noodles at hand, substitute whole-wheat linguini. If gluten is a problem, try the nut sauce on gluten-free pasta or zucchini "pasta" made using a vegetable peeler or spiral slicer.

Preparation: Combine the almond butter, rice vinegar, tamari, honey, garlic, ginger, water, sea salt, and cayenne pepper in a blender. Process until smooth. Bring a pot of lightly salted water to a boil. Add the soba noodles and cook 1 to 2 minutes if the noodles are fresh or 5 to 6 minutes if the noodles are dried. Drain in a colander. Put the noodles into a serving dish and toss with the sauce and chopped scallions. Makes 2 servings as a main dish, 4 as a side dish.

Ingredients:

Sauce:
2 tbsp organic almond butter
2 tbsp rice vinegar
1½ tbsp tamari or coconut aminos
1 tbsp raw, local honey
2 garlic cloves, chopped
3 tbsp minced fresh ginger
2 tbsp water
sea salt to taste
cayenne pepper to taste

Noodles:
1/4 lb soba noodles
1/2 c chopped scallions

Farmers' Market Vegetable Soup

I make this soup throughout the year, but I like it best in the winter, when I can toss in lots of root vegetables and dark leafy greens for a rich and warming supper dish. The soup changes with the seasons; the one constant is the mirepoix base. In French cuisine, the classic mirepoix of chopped carrots, onions, and celery is used to provide an aromatic base to a soup. Kombu, a type of Japanese seaweed, is a great addition to this or any soup. It deepens the flavors and adds a slightly salty, savory taste. Be creative with this recipe—make it with whatever looks freshest and most enticing at the farmers' market that day. Just be sure to always include at least 1 cup of dark leafy greens, such as kale, spinach, or collards.

Preparation: Heat the olive oil in a large soup pot over medium heat. Add the carrot, onion, celery, garlic, and leek. Cook, stirring often, until the vegetables are softened but not browned, about 4 to 5 minutes. Add the tomatoes, parsley, basil, thyme, kombu, bay leaf, red pepper flakes, and vegetable stock. Season to taste with sea salt. Bring the mixture to a boil and add the vegetables. Simmer the soup for about 1 hour, or until all the vegetables are tender. Add the dark leafy greens and cook for 5 minutes longer. Makes about 8 servings.

Ingredients:

2 tsp extra-virgin olive oil
1 small carrot, diced
1/2 onion, diced
1/2 stalk celery, diced
4 garlic cloves, minced
1 leek, cut into thin rounds
2 c organic tomatoes
1/2 c coarsely chopped parsley
2 tbsp chopped fresh basil or 1 tsp dried
1 tsp fresh thyme leaves or 1/2 tsp dried
1 4-in piece kombu
1 bay leaf
1 tsp red pepper flakes
8 c organic vegetable stock
sea salt to taste
4 c assorted seasonal vegetables, cut into small pieces
1 c dark leafy greens, sliced into thin ribbons

Ingredients:

2 acorn or kabocha squash
1 c wild rice
4 c water
1 to 2 tsp sea salt
2 onions
1 c precooked chestnuts
1 to 2 c mushrooms (any
  kind or a mixture)
2 c dark leafy greens,
  shredded (any kind or a
  mixture)
1 to 2 tbsp coconut oil
black pepper to taste

Wild Rice and Chestnut Stuffed Acorn Squash Bowl

Dr. Alejandro Junger is the bestselling author of *Clean* and *Clean Gut*. He's a cardiologist and an expert on restoring your body's natural ability to heal itself. Dr. Junger has shared this recipe created by Jenny Nelson, his wellness chef. She creates the wonderful recipes found at his website, cleanprogram.com. Roasted winter squash, stuffed with a medley of wild rice, richly flavored chestnuts, and vegetables, is perfect for every Nutritional Style. This rich vegetarian dish is so satisfying that meat lovers will never notice that it has no animal foods in it. Precooked chestnuts are usually sold in jars; look for them in the gourmet section of your supermarket.

Preparation: Preheat oven to 400°F. Carefully slice off the top quarter of each squash, keeping the stem in place. Set the tops aside. Place the squashes, cut-side down, on a baking sheet and bake until just tender all the way through, about 20 to 30 minutes. Add the stemmed tops halfway through the cooking time. While the squashes cook, prepare the wild rice. In a saucepan, bring 4 c of water with 1 tsp sea salt to a boil. Add the wild rice and stir gently. When the water returns to a boil, reduce the heat to low and partially cover the pot with a lid, leaving a 1-inch crack for steam to escape. Simmer until the liquid is absorbed and the wild rice is tender, about 30 to 45 minutes, depending on how soft you like it. Roughly chop the onions, chestnuts, and mushrooms. In a large pan over medium heat, melt the coconut oil. Add the onions and chestnuts and cook, stirring frequently, until tender and brown. Add the wild rice, mushrooms, and greens and continue to cook, stirring often, until everything is slightly browned and crispy. Season to taste with sea salt and black pepper. To prepare the squashes, scoop out and discard the seeds. Fill the squashes with the wild rice and vegetable mixture, packing it in tightly. Cover the stuffed squashes with the tops. Return the squashes to the oven and bake until very soft and browned, about 30 minutes longer. To serve, place both squashes on a serving platter. Cut them into halves or quarters at the table. Makes 4 servings.

Resources

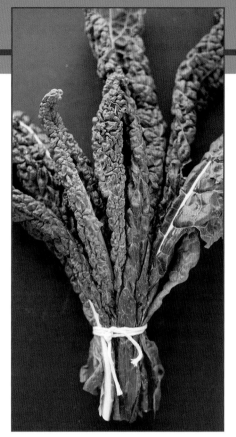

I value my go-to online resources—they're where I find information and inspiration (beyond what I get from my clients). When someone recommends a valuable new site or I track one down myself, it can make my day. A reliable, accurate source for food, recipes, knowledge, restaurants, skin care, boutique companies that sell in a responsible way and use organic ingredients—that rings my chimes.

The resources below are my top faves, the virtual emporiums and accurate information sources I find myself returning to often. Sadly, however, I don't have space to list all the sites I find helpful. My full list is an ever-changing collection of goodies, and I'm always on the hunt. To see an up-to-date list of resources, including physical places, my favorite books, and more, check my website at hollithompson.com. Be sure to sign up for my weekly updates, where I blog about the latest and greatest. If you're really into knowing everything that I know, follow me on Facebook, Twitter, Pinterest, and Instagram. No kidding, I'm nonstop.

Friends with Holistic Benefits

ewg.org
Features the Environmental Working Groups' guides to clean cosmetics, household cleaning products, sunscreens, safe produce, and more.

lesscancer.org
Founder Bill Couzens is an early advocate for cancer prevention; this site is a resource for cancer prevention and risk reduction.

mindbodygreen.com
A daily update with interesting and informative articles on nutrition, health, and the environment.

thedailylove.com
Founder Mastin Kipp is a next-generation spirit seeker. His daily blog features posts from well-known advocates of a healthy lifestyle.

Essential Oils

doterra.com
My go-to place for essential oils. I love their products and integrity. They offer home products, body care, and supplements, too. I adore their On Guard Cleaner for my home and Deep Blue rub for after intense workouts.

Water You Want to Drink

aquaovo.com
Limoges china water filters; glass water bottles in stylish designs

Friends with Nutritional How-To

bewellbydrfranklipman.com
Dr. Frank Lipman's site for high-quality cleanse kits, guidelines, recipes, and supplements.

cleanprogram.com
Dr. Alejandro Junger's site for his detox program, support, and recipes.

detoxtheworld.com
Natalia Rose is a leader in the detox movement and the best-selling author of *Forever Beautiful*. Her site has lots of information to offer.

drhyman.com
Dr. Mark Hyman's blog, recipes, and supportive community are a consistent resource.

kriscarr.com
Kris is a cancer survivor, speaker, author, and a great lady. She shares weekly on nutrition and lifestyle, and she loves her doggies, too.

oneluckyduck.com
Raw food guru Sarma Melngailis offers an inspirational blog. You can also learn about and order her great products.

Eat (and Drink) Well

celiac.org
Resources and information for people with celiac disease.

eatwellguide.org
An on-line guide that offers resources, maps, and directories for locally grown, sustainable food in the United States and Canada.

farmersmarket.com
Type in your locale or Zip code and find the nearest farmers' market.

happyherbalist.com
A great resource for all things herbal—a little hippie looking and fun to read. Good source for kombucha starter kits.

localharvest.org
Locate farmers' markets and purveyors of organic and sustainable food nationwide.

meatlessmonday.com
Support and inspiration for meatless Monday meals with a focus on family. Going meatless on Monday (more often if you can) is a great way to help the environment while helping your health.

pressedjuicedirectory.com
Founder Max Goldberg follows the pressed juice trend closely. Search here to find organic juice in your area and for raw food and juice delivery.

seafoodwatch.org
Use this site for up-to-date information about safe and sustainable seafood.

Boutique Food Companies

babycakesnyc.com
Delicious cupcakes and baked treats without common intolerance triggers such as dairy, gluten, and white sugar. Yes, I said delicious.

bellocq.com
Bespoke, organic teas in stylish packaging. These make the perfect hostess gift.

crownmaple.com
Organic maple syrup that comes in a streamlined, handsome bottle; enough to encourage your granola-making every week.

raakachocolate.com
Made by hand in Brooklyn, these bars are creative, exotic, and organic, too. Try the coconut milk bar, or the chocolate of the month club, with offerings like Camino Verde, Ecuador, or Bourbon Cask Aged.

savannahbee.com
You'll want to order everything on this site. Local honey from the Savannah area offers a variety of flavors. The wildflower honey makes me smile, with notes of white holly and saw palmetto. Their body products are fabulous, too, and they even offer something that soothes puppy dog paws.

sunfood.com
The quality of superfoods, nuts, and seeds at Sunfood is reliably excellent. The cashews are to die for.

tinybutmightyfoods.com
Tiny but Mighty popcorn is the best ever. You can rest assured that it's not GMO, unlike most of the corn in our country. Try sprinkling with a little EVOO and sea salt.

vosgeschocolate.com
Luckily, these chocolates are becoming more widely distributed, because they are amazing. Check out their dark chocolate and superfood collection.

Feel Beautiful

acureorganics.com
My yoga trainer swears by this skin-care line, as do many clients.

alkaitis.com
This company goes by the motto, "If you can't eat it, don't put it on your skin." I love that.

annmariegianni.com
Organic, natural, and wild-crafted skin care; beloved by many of my colleagues.

eminenceorganics.com
A celebrity favorite, this organic skin care company from Hungary uses biodynamic ingredients.

juicebeauty.com
Reasonably priced skin care that's organic and clean; their packaging is, too. I love their lip gloss and daily skin care lines.

lilamae.com
This site sells only products made in the United States. You can find some fabulous organic skin care here (also gorgeous home entertaining pieces).

mychelle.com
My personal favorite is the eyelash conditioner, and a friend swears by the Pure Harmony Cleanser, Mist and Cream. Some men I know love their products, too.

onehundredpercentpure.com
A favorite of mine, my clients, and my friends for years. Favorites are their Organic Coffee Bean Caffeine Eye Cream and Nourishing Body Lotions. We love all their scents!

shopolivine.com
Addictive organic fragrances with names like "More Than the Stars" and "Full Regalia"; there's no worry here about harmful chemicals in your fragrance.

sukiskincare.com
A luxury skin-care line with a celebrity following; known to deliver beautiful results.

tataharper.com
A Vermont brand with a cult following, this is a sure bet.

vapourbeauty.com
Clean makeup with on-trend colors and wonderful texture. I adore their foundation and eye shadows. They're one of my favorites.

Get Moving

barre3.com
This is fitness that matches my style. Great barre classes taught in a real-life kind of way. Baby in the kitchen, anyone?

gaiamtv.com
A wonderful resource for yoga instruction videos and mind/body inspiration videos.

tracyandersonmethod.com
Anderson's site is elegant and devoted to holistic health. Her movement program has a strong dance component. It's challenging, but you'll get results. And Gwyneth Paltrow is now partnering with her.

xenstrengthyoga.com
Danielle Diamond created her own style of yoga, designed for maximum efficiency and effectiveness and using weights for extra toning. Xen Strength suits her Manhattan celebrity clients just fine. You can download workouts on the go if you can't catch her live.

yogaglo.com
Yoga videos that suit everyone at every level, featuring all styles of yoga movement. Yogis follow this site with a passion.

Ready to Study Nutrition?

integrativenutrition.com
Earn your certification as a health coach in this popular virtual program that offers many live components. Offers a strong business and coaching component as well. Vist hollithompson.com for my personal story about this amazing school.

cnhp.org
Earn your certified natural health practitioner certification in this holistic program. Courses are available online and in locations nationwide.

ecornell.com/certificates/plant-based-nutrition/certificate-in-plant-based-nutrition/
A virtual course from Cornell University, based on Professor Emeritus T. Colin Campbell's bestselling book, *The China Study.*

My Go-Tos for Recipe Inspiration

Food52.com
One of my favorite foodie sites, they offer recipes and helpful how-tos. Their provisions section makes me drool; I want all of it for my kitchen. Many recipes to choose from. Check out their kombucha and kimchi kits.

goop.com
I'm a raving fan of Gwyneth Paltrow and all that she's up to. She delivers weekly inspiration at this site, elegantly served up in a stylish way.

greenkitchenstories.com
Winner of the best food blog, this site is loaded with creative ideas and healthy recipes.

mynewroots.com
Chef Sarah Britton's site is deliciously lovely; I aspire some day to cook half as well as she does.

naturallyella.com
The motto here is: be healthy, eat delicious. If you glance through this site, you'll never want to leave.

101cookbooks.com
Chef Heidi Swanson satisfies my love of food and creative cooking, in a healthy way. Her cookbooks are my favorites, too; they always deliver recipes I can count on.

smittenkitchen.com
I love this site's seasonal approach to eating. The beautiful photographs capture what I want to create in my own kitchen.

thekindlife.com
Alicia Silverstone reminds me why nutrition is a priority in my life. Her site is easy on the eyes and I always learn something new.

Index

during autumn and winter, 138–140
during cancer treatments, 82, 84, 85
during cleanse, 66, 69, 71–72

K

Kale (autumn superfood), 137
Kombu (year-round superfood), 175
Kombucha (year-round superfood), 175

L

Lactose intolerance, 38–39
Lavender, 164–165
Leafy greens (spring superfood), 93
Legumes during cleansing, 68
Liquid nutrition during cleanse, 71–72
Living foods, 72

M

Maca powder (year-round superfood), 175
Magnesium, 164
Metabolism boosters, 135–136
Minerals in cleansing baths, 100
Mineral supplements during winter, 161, 164
Modern Vegans, 13–15
    cleanse for
        eating out during, 76
        liquid nutrition during, 71
        protocol, 74
        raw foods during, 72
    creamy soup for, 192
    snacks, 191
    soy and, 41–42
    sweets for, 188
Moodiness. *See* Irritability
Mothers and weight obsessions, 26
Movement. *See* Exercise
Mucus production, 37–38
Mystery foods, 51–52

N

Nausea, 136
Noncaloric sugar substitutes, 45, 53–56
Nondairy milk/creamers during prep for cleansing, 67
Nutmeg, 136
Nutrient absorption and gluten, 34
Nutrition
    consequences of poor, 2–4, 17
    healing and, 83–86
    importance of proper, 4–5
    web resources for information, 202, 206

Nutritional style
    adapting your, 17–19, 21
    consequences of improper, 2–4, 17, 18, 19
    finding your, 10–11, 20–23
    raw foods and, 108–110
    uniqueness of each individual's, 8
Nutritional yeast (year-round superfood), 175
Nuts (year-round superfood), 69, 175

O

Oils, essential, 100–101
Oils and fats during cleansing, 68
Omnivores, 8–9
    See also Healthy Omnivores
1–2–1 cleansing schedule, 64–65
Organic foods
    dairy products, 40
    gluten-free, 36
    processed, 51–52
    produce, 49–51
    soy, 42–53
Osteoporosis, 40

P

Persimmons (winter superfood), 158
Pesticides, 49–51
PH theory and winter foods, 157
Phytoestrogens, 42
Phytonutrients, 85
Pomegranates (autumn superfood), 137
Pressed juices, 139, 203
Probiotics, 140–141
Processed foods
    dangers in, 51–52
    during prep and cleansing, 65, 67
    electrolyte balance and, 115
    prevalence of, 91, 92–93
    sugar in, 43
Protein
    during winter, 155
    sources for raw food diet, 110
    See also Animal protein
Puffy eyes, cleansing to reduce, 63–64
Pumpkin (autumn superfood), 137

Q

Quinoa (year-round superfood), 155, 176
Quiz for finding your nutritional style, 10–11